Noshe___ ___rthore

CREDIT CARD SALE

76045   EXP: 8325   8325

MC EXP DATE: 0304
MC AUTH#
07199A
MC #
512107500294507A

CHANGE	0.00
MASTER CARD	10.65
TOTAL	10.65
6.500% TAX	0.65
SUBTOTAL	10.00

31050400009 Short Sleeve	0.00	TX
31637700007 Misc Sleepwear	10.00	TX

07:43PM   06 MAY 2002

27BHAWTHORN CENTRE
LIMBO LOUNGE

SALES FINAL

LIMBO LOUNGE
?THAWTHORN CENTRE

31S37780007 Misc Sleepwear 10.00 TX
31054080009 Short Sleeve 0.00 TX
SUBTOTAL 10.00
6.5000% TAX 0.65
TOTAL 10.65
MASTER CARD 10.65
CHANGE 0.00

MC # 512107500294507?
MC AUTH# 071594
MC EXP DATE: 0304

ALL SALES FINAL

CREDIT CARD SALE

CUSTOMER COPY

THE WAR WITHIN US

Everyman's guide to infection and immunity

Cedric Mims

Emeritus Professor
Department of Microbiology
Guy's Hospital Medical School
London, UK

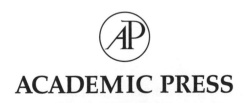

ACADEMIC PRESS

A Harcourt Science and Technology Company

San Diego   San Francisco   New York
Boston   London   Sydney   Tokyo

Academic Press
A Harcourt Science and Technology Company
Harcourt Place, 32 Jamestown Road, London NW1 7BY, UK
http://www.academicpress.com

Academic Press
A Harcourt Science and Technology Company
525 B Street, Suite 1900, San Diego, California 92101-4495, USA
http://www.academicpress.com

ISBN 0-12-498251-4

A catalogue record for this book is available from the British Library

Printed and bound in Great Britain by MPG Books Ltd, Cornwall, UK

00 01 02 03 04 05 MP 9 8 7 6 5 4 3 2 1

CONTENTS

ACKNOWLEDGEMENTS

The book was begun during a one-month stay as a writer in residence at the Bellagio Study and Conference Center, Bellagio, Italy. It was a wonderful place for work and for thought, in the company of scholars from other disciplines, other countries. I am grateful to the Rockefeller Foundation for giving me that opportunity. I am also grateful to my microbiological colleagues over the past 45 years for their unconscious contributions to this book, and to John Sheaff for his tutorials on word-processing. Above all I must thank Vicky Mims for her loving support and for her patience in reading and constructively criticizing the manuscript.

PREFACE

Many of the ideas expressed here have been developed also by others. The concept of an infectious disease as the result of an armed conflict between parasite and host, in which strategies and counterstrategies are employed, was a feature of an earlier book, *The Pathogenesis of Infectious Disease*, first published in 1976.

It can be tiresome to be told something one already knows and equally tiresome to be expected to know what one does not know. There is no solution to this, and I can do no more than mention the problem as I chart a course through Nature's ways. In making the intricacies of the immune system and infectious diseases less baffling to the general reader I have had to simplify, filter the facts, and give phenomena a purpose. I make no apologies for this. Nor do I apologize for taking the reader some way into the intricacies of modern immunology; and the first three parts of the book are especially for those who like to know *how* and *why*.

Tales of wonderbugs, wonderdrugs, death and contagion are regular news items, and we have all suffered from and been vaccinated against infectious diseases, but there is widespread ignorance about such matters. We do not need to know how a car or a television set works when we use it, but I believe that some understanding of how the body responds to microbial invaders is worthwhile. After all, it happens inside every one of us, regularly, and is a personal, intimate affair. Surely we owe it to our own bodies to be interested?

INTRODUCTION

Supposing you are a creature that has decided to take up parasitism. You are fed up with the hardships and uncertainties of the outside world and seek the protection of life inside another creature's body. At first sight it seems an easy enough option. Free board and lodging, no need for that constant search for food, no need to watch out at all times for danger, or to withstand harsh climates.

What do you have to do? The rules are the same, however small you are. First, having chosen your host, you have to stick onto its body or get inside it. Then you have to grow, increase your numbers, and finally leave the body so that some of your descendants can invade other bodies and carry on with the cycle. If you don't manage to do these things your species will die out and become extinct.

But when you look at it more closely it is not such an easy matter. Your possible hosts have been faced with this threat for millions of years and have developed powerful armour and equipped themselves with lethal weapons to repel and kill invaders. The warm, inviting body turns out to be a basically hostile one, and if you are to survive as a parasite you have to get round the defences. The penalty for failure is death.

This is why the story of parasitism is one of armed conflict, a war in which the defences of the host have called forth answering strategies by the parasite, which have led in turn to counterstrategies on the part of the host. The ancient conflict has been going on since life began, and it means that parasitism is no easy way out from the hazards that you face as a free-living creature. A new set of hazards await you once you get inside.

Nevertheless of the millions of different species on the earth, almost as many have opted for the parasitic as for the free-living way of life. Long ago the English playwright Ben Jonson (1572–1637) noted that

> *'Almost*
> *All the wise world is little else in Nature*
> *But parasites or sub-parasites'*
> (from Volpone, 1606)

All creatures, whether crabs, trees, jellyfish, frogs, roses, elephants, coconuts, bacteria or humans, have their parasites, and they are hard to get rid of. Think of the human species, which at this stage in its evolution has eliminated its competitors, but not its parasites. The parasites remain important causes of disease in most of us, and so far we have been unable to get rid of them. I include in the category of parasites everything from a virus, by definition a parasite of living cells, to a large parasite like a tapeworm. Naturally the parasite is smaller than the host, and in this book the main focus is on the smallest ones of all, the microbes, so-called because they are visible only under the microscope.

Human beings are host to about 1500 different microbes, and you, dear reader, have already encountered several hundred of them. Like all parasites, they have to tread carefully. If they cause too much damage their own future is at risk. They should do what they have to do, and do it as unobtrusively as possible. They should enter your body, warding off your attack while they multiply, and then leave without causing serious illness. Most of our 1500 microbes are harmless, but about 100 of them are not so well-behaved and can make you ill during their stay in the body. It can be anything from a trivial inconvenience to a life-threatening disease. The viruses that cause skin warts or common colds, like the microbes that spend their lives in your mouth and bowels, give little or no trouble. Influenza and measles, on the other hand, make you ill, and HIV and rabies are deadly.

Doctors and patients, of course, are more interested in the ones that make you ill, and news items tell us about wonderbugs and wonderdrugs, and about plagues, contagion, and death. Books and movies have the same preoccupation. In this book, however, we shall see that the harmless invader often tell a more subtle, intriguing story.

Surprisingly few of us understand how our bodies defend us and do battle against invaders, and how the invaders occasionally cause disease. As it happens, the last ten years have seen an explosion in knowledge about these matters, exciting for the man in the street as well as for the scientists.

The hows and whys of infectious disease make a fascinating story with implications for all of us during the 21st century.

This book is an account of the ancient war between the invader and the defender, between the microbial parasite and the host. It is basically a military account, although we shall see that the invader behaves more like a spy in foreign territory than a soldier. We will often take his point of view. In going about his business inside our body he must use the utmost ingenuity, knowing that we are armed to the teeth and that death lurks round every corner. Should we not admire the resourcefulness and cunning of the invaders that have made a success of it?

Yet if we complained to a committee of microbes, accusing them of causing us such a burden of suffering, we might get a surprising answer. You go on about us being parasites, they could say, but in fact it is you who are parasitic on us! Without us the whole of plant and animal life on the earth would collapse. Those of us who live in the roots of plants like clover and capture nitrogen from the air help with the essential recycling of life's elements. Others of us spend our lives breaking down and disposing of dead plants and animals. Without us, mountains of rotting material would accumulate on the surface of the earth. We also dispose of your body wastes, and would like to point out that your sewage works could not function without us. And what about the cows, rabbits, termites and other animals that need us to digest their food and owe their very existence to us? As an extra bonus we add to your quality of life, by enabling you to make bread, cheeses, beers and wines. Even your oil was formed by the action of us microbes millions of years ago. Admittedly a few have taken advantage of your comfortable bodies and made their homes there, but surely the overall picture is one of humans being dependent and in a real sense parasitic on us microbes!

Part 1

THE PARASITE VERSUS THE HOST

Chapter 1

THE PARASITE VERSUS THE HOST

PARASITISM AS A WAY OF LIFE

'I keep six honest serving men
(They taught me all I knew);
Their names are What and Why and When
And How and Where and Who.'
Just So Stories (1902)
'The Elephants Child'
Rudyard Kipling (1865-1936).

This book is about parasites. They live in or on their hosts, and while a few are quite large (tapeworm), most are microscopically small (microbes such as viruses and bacteria). There are good and there are bad parasites. They range from unobtrusive more or less harmless ones to virulent invaders that cause severe sickness or death. Let us consider some examples to show the spectrum of possibilities.

Stephanie's skin worries

Stephanie, aged 15, lives in Bristol, England, and is worried about her skin. For some months there have been ugly red spots on her forehead and shoulders, and they aren't made much better by the ointments and creams she buys from the chemist. And lately she has the feeling that her body has an unpleasant smell. What is going on?

The skin protects us from the outside world, and takes a regular buffeting. To cope with this, it constantly renews itself from below. In the bottommost layers the skin cells divide, pushing up their progeny towards the surface. As they move up they get thinner, flatter, eventually die and are shed from the body as tiny skin flakes. We lose more than a million each day, and a veritable shower is released when we undress. The fine layer of white dust that your finger picks up from the top of a shelf or cupboard consists mostly of dead skin cells. In this way your skin is completely replaced every week or so.

The dry outer layers have to be kept moist and supple, and a layer of oily material oozes out over the skin from tens of thousands of tiny sebaceous glands (Latin, *sebum* = grease) that open onto the surface. Stephanie's problem is that she is undergoing the changes of adolescence. Sex hormones are transforming her into a woman but they are also causing overactivity of the sebaceous glands. The glands get blocked, and the resident bacteria on the skin, which are normally harmless parasites, grow in the blocked glands and form substances that give rise to inflammation and redness. She is convinced she looks terrible, and cannot understand why she has to suffer while her friend Joan has such clear unblemished skin. Finally the GP starts her on a long course of antibiotics to keep the bacteria out of the glands, and things get a bit better. But the acne spots may stay until she has 'grown out of it' in her early twenties.

The worry that she smells is part of the general feeling that she is unattractive, but once again the resident skin bacteria have something to answer for. When her sweat and the oily secretions from the sebaceous glands first arrive at the skin surface they do not smell unpleasant. Resident bacteria, however, use these secretions as food and form odoriferous products, especially in the armpits. Luckily, most deodorants act against these particular bacteria, and this problem is solved without difficulty.

Stephanie's skin bacteria can be looked on as well-behaved parasites as long as they don't harm her, but they overstepped the mark when they contributed to her acne.

Mark has bad teeth

Stephanie's younger brother Mark has a different problem. His skin is clear but he is a regular visitor at the dentist and is always having new fillings. Although he is supposed to brush his teeth twice a day and go easy on sweets, he doesn't keep to this and his mother is tired of nagging him. At this rate he will have false teeth by the time he is grown up. What is going on in his mouth?

The resident microbes in most people's mouths include a certain bacterium called *Streptococcus mutans*, which is nicely adapted to life on teeth. It is able to stick firmly to teeth, grows to establish a colony, and various other microbes take advantage of this by joining the colony, so that the whole thing forms a thin film of multiplying organisms called a dental plaque. Under the microscope this patch on the tooth looks like a tangled forest, perfectly placed to make use of the nutrients present in the mouth. If you remove it by brushing it re-establishes itself in a few hours. *S. mutans* loves sugar and flourishes when it is regularly available. Unfortunately acid is formed from the sugar, and if the plaque is not removed regularly, the acid bores a small hole in the enamel. The hole gets bigger, exposing the sensitive layers under the enamel, and Mark gets another toothache. If he brushed more often and stopped eating sweets between meals, it wouldn't be so bad. But without the bacteria the tooth-rot (caries) could not develop in the first place. Indeed caries can be regarded as an infectious disease, one of the commonest in the modern world. With our frequently sugary diet we are especially vulnerable. Having strong enamel helps, and although Mark is unlikely to be deficient in fluoride, it could be that he has inherited some genes that make him susceptible. As in the case of Stephanie's skin microbes, the residents in Mark's mouth have ceased to be harmless guests and have done some damage.

Both Stephanie and Mark have had threadworms

I should add that both Stephanie and Mark have encountered a very successful parasitic worm. When they were 4–5 years old they attended a preschool three mornings a week, and it was there that eggs of the human threadworm or pinworm (*Enterobius vermicularis*) found their way into their mouths. The eggs hatched, and in their intestines grew into the threadlike adult worms. The worms (about fifty of them), each only about a centimetre long, enjoyed a comfortable life, surrounded by plenty of food. They did no damage to the intestinal wall and managed to stay put without being carried along and expelled in the stools. Stephanie and Mark were none the worse for being the unwitting hosts. But, like all parasites, the threadworm has to make its way to fresh hosts if it is to survive. To achieve this it has an ingenious strategy. At night, when the children are quiet in bed, the adult female worm, laden with thousands of eggs, makes its way down the intestine to the anus, sticks out its rear end, and, feeling its way, deposits its eggs onto the skin round the anus. The wriggly movements of the worm cause itching. The children then scratch their bottoms vigorously, and in doing so pick up the eggs under their fingernails. And unwashed or poorly washed hands are fine vehicles for transferring the eggs to the fingers and mouths of other children.

The worm is easily eliminated by drugs but it generally causes no other symptoms, and children recover without treatment. If necessary the doctor can make the diagnosis by pressing a piece of sellotape onto the skin round the anus and then removing it and identifying the typical tiny eggs under the microscope. The human threadworm is a highly successful parasite, infecting millions of children, and doing little or no damage. This is more than can be said for many less well-behaved parasitic worms, such as hookworms, tapeworms, and those that cause schistosomiasis and elephantiasis.

So far, Stephanie and Mark have met only the gentlest parasites. Later in life they will catch influenza, glandular fever, and one or two other unpleasant diseases. Luckily they have been vaccinated against many of them, including whooping cough, tetanus, polio, measles and diphtheria, and are fortunate to live in a country where there is no malaria, leprosy, cholera, typhoid or yellow fever. When they read in the paper about bubonic plague, Ebola or rabies, which are life-threatening infections in Africa and India, they realize they are in a safe country, and better off than Ricardo, even though his life was not actually threatened.

Ricardo will stay small

Ricardo is three years old, and his parents are poor. It is 1976, and he lives in a village in Guatemala where there is no sewage disposal, the drinking water is contaminated, and the nearest doctor 25 miles away. Luckily he had been vaccinated against tetanus, diphtheria and polio. Until he was born his body was sterile and free of microbes and then, during the first few weeks of life, a host of friendly microbes colonized his skin, mouth and intestines, and became regular residents. This is what happens to us all. But in his family and in his village he is surrounded by less benevolent ones awaiting the opportunity to invade. For a month or two the antibodies in his mother's milk protected him, but then, as he breathed the air from people's coughs and sneezes and his diet began to include the local water and food, the other microbial parasites found their opportunity.

At four and a half months of age he suffered two attacks of diarrhoea and a chest infection, and by the time he was 18 months old there had been another eight episodes of diarrhoea, each caused by a different intestinal invader, each one making him fret for a few days and lose a bit of weight. Catching measles at nine months was a major setback; it was yet another nutritional handicap and it took him a month to get over it. Several attacks of bronchitis added to the burden. Then three different parasitic worms took up residence in his intestines. It was a disastrous first year, and now his weight showed little increase because every few weeks new microbes found their way into his small body. He suffered from impetigo, thrush, conjunctivitis, a severe middle ear infection, and more diarrhoea.

Ricardo is a lively and cheerful child, but at three years he weighs only nine and a half kilograms, less than two-thirds of the weight of a three-year-old in a Western country blessed with clean water, sewage disposal, medicines, and doctors. In his short life he has been host to 63 different microbial parasites. Although he had fought them off and cleared most of them from his body, the battles had left their mark and he will never grow to be as big as he might have been.

But that is how it was for most of the children in his village. The picture was one of heavy pressure from parasites, with the scales tipped heavily in their favour. It has been the pattern in settled communities all over the world for thousands of years. Ricardo's life would have been transformed by the clean water, sewage disposal, better diet, medicines and vaccines enjoyed by Stephanie and Mark. But these things cost money. He was a victim, and the parasites reaped the benefit, exploiting his small sad body. Since then things have improved in his village, but elsewhere in the world there are children who continue to suffer as Ricardo did.

Rajam's unfortunate meeting with a dog

Rajam, aged 12, represents the final stage in the parasite spectrum. He lived in a small village in Southern India, and loved animals. While visiting his aunt in a nearby village he had stroked a dog that looked sad and lost, and it gave him a small nip on the left hand for his trouble. Two months later Rajam became unwell with fever, headache and nausea. It didn't seem much, but his left hand began to hurt, and the following week he had some muscle spasms in the arm, then a convulsion. He got worse and his parents began to despair, but nothing could be done. Finally he went into a coma and died.

The disease was rabies, caused by a virus, one of the smallest parasites. It infects animals such as dogs, cats, foxes, jackals, wolves, skunks, raccoons and vampire bats, and keeps itself going in these animals by growing in their salivary glands and spreading from animal to animal by biting and licking. There can be a hundred thousand doses of virus in every drop of saliva. Rabies is common in India, and the dog that gave Rajam that bite was infected. The disease can be prevented by a vaccine, but once you have become sick it is too late.

Some parasites are useful

The stories of Ricardo and Rajam illustrate the worst features of parasitism. Sometimes it is not such a one-way process, and the host actually derives some benefit from the invader. Take the microbes that have colonized and live in the stomach (rumen) of cows, or in the intestine (caecum) of rabbits. These animals cannot digest cellulose, which is the main food item in leaves and grasses. The microbes in their intestines, however, are able to do this. They supply the host with the nutrients they have formed from cellulose, and at the same time they enjoy food and shelter. The rumen of a 500 kg cow is a complex fermentation chamber, housing 17 different species of bacteria, which provide food for at least seven types of protozoa. As these swarming microbes multiply the surplus is shunted through to the intestine to be killed, digested and absorbed. In the process large volumes of carbon dioxide and methane are formed and expelled from both ends of the cow. Things are slightly more complicated for the rabbit, because the place where the microbes live, the appendix, is further down the intestine, beyond the part where food is absorbed. To solve this problem the rabbit recycles its faeces. Soft white pellets are formed during the daytime and the rabbit eats them, so that the digested food can be absorbed. At night the pellets are the familiar brown ones, deposited on the grass for us to see. Without the microbes the cows and the rabbits would die of starvation. We call this symbiosis or mutualism. Both the host and the parasite benefit.

The microbes living in the human intestines are in a different category. They too receive free food, board and lodging, and they are parasites, yet most of the time we are neither worse nor better off for having them. However, as regular residents, each with its own special territory in the intestine, they tend to keep out less-pleasant invaders. If you kill them off with antibiotics you may suffer intrusions by microbes such as *Candida* and develop thrush. Also they form certain vitamins, which can be useful if you are starved of these vitamins. So parasitism sometimes merges into symbiosis.

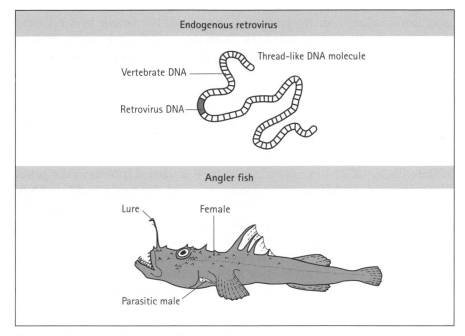

Figure 1 Two extraordinary parasites.

We have seen that for the host, parasitism comes in a variety of forms. It can be so mild as to be unnoticed, it can cause an unpleasant disease, or it can be lethal. Before we leave our consideration of parasitism as a way of life, let us consider two extraordinary examples (Figure 1), just to show the great range of possibilities.

Angler fish – a message for the human race?

Angler fish (*Ceratioidea* species) live deep down in the dark recesses of the oceans, so deep that they rarely encounter any life, let alone a member of the opposite sex. They have adapted to this lonely life by having an angler's lure, sometimes illuminated, projecting from the top of the head to attract prey, plus an enormous mouth and stomach to handle the largest of food items. For many years all the angler fish described by zoologists were females; there was no record of a male. However, just behind the gill slit is a tiny knob, about 1/1000th of the size of the female. Astonishingly, this proved to be the male! It is a total parasite, obtaining all nutrients from the female. With no requirement for fins, intestines, brain, eyes, and so on, these organs have disappeared and the male has been reduced to his essence, his only justification, a sperm-producing sac. When the female lays her eggs the sperm are discharged over them. Strictly speaking the relationship is symbiotic because the female benefits by having such a convenient supply of sperm.

Endogenous retroviruses – the perfect parasites

So that you can appreciate these retroviruses, the perfect parasites, I need to remind you of the ABC of molecular biology. In nearly all living creatures the normal pathway of biological information in terms of molecules is from DNA to RNA to protein. Information is carried (*coded*) in the genes (DNA, the material of inheritance) and is converted (*transcribed*) into RNA, which then *translates* the message into proteins (enzymes, cell-building materials, etc.). Viruses are unique because their genetic information can be carried in either DNA or RNA. There are DNA viruses and there are RNA viruses. Retroviruses give an extra twist to the story because their genetic information is coded in the form of RNA, but when they multiply this RNA is first converted (transcribed) back into DNA, which is the reverse of the usual process. This is why they are called retroviruses (Latin, *retro* = backward). HIV is our most famous retrovirus.

Furthermore, when these retroviruses multiply in host cells their freshly formed DNA is inserted directly into the genes (DNA molecules) of the host. The infected cell now carries a foreign passenger in the form of retrovirus DNA. If the cell divides, the descendant cells will also carry the passenger. If the infected cell is a reproductive cell (sperm cell, egg cell) the retrovirus DNA will be in the fertilized egg and will be handed down to all cells of the offspring. The retrovirus DNA is not recognized as a foreigner, yet it is nevertheless a parasite. It has become part of the inheritance. As long as it does no harm it is watched over, protected, and duplicated indefinitely, as if it were the host's own DNA. HIV, thank goodness, does not behave in this way.

It turns out that over the course of hundreds of millions of years of evolution, very large numbers of retroviruses have inserted themselves into the DNA of vertebrate animals. In humans at least 3% of the total DNA is of this type. These retroviruses are securely established in the host species and are referred to as 'endogenous'. There is no need for such parasites to spread to fresh hosts, no need for infectious forms, because the parasite is present in everyone. Accordingly, their DNA is now incapable of producing infectious virus material and they can be looked upon as 'retroviral fossils'. This is surely the ultimate, the final and logical step in parasitism! Get inside the genes of the host. The DNA of the retrovirus is perfectly placed. In the final analysis all nature cares about is the handing down of DNA (genes) from one generation to the next, and indeed we can look upon our bodies, our very lives on earth, as no more than devices used by human DNA to ensure its survival. From this point of view all DNA is selfish, and the DNA of a retrovirus as selfish as any other. In some ways retroviruses are equivalent to computer viruses, insofar as they get into the hard disc (host DNA) where they proliferate and maintain themselves simply because they know how to.

BUT PARASITES HAVE PROBLEMS

Obviously parasites enjoy many advantages. Those that live actually inside the host are protected from the outside world and have all their nutrients supplied by the host. This means that more resources can be given over to multiplication and reproduction. Also, because they are cut off from the outside world there is no need for ordinary sense organs like eyes and ears, as long as they develop acute awareness of their chemical surroundings inside the host. It is by responding to chemical cues that they know where they are in the body, when to switch on this or that protection against the host's attack, when to start multiplying (Box 1). On the whole it seems like an easy life, warm, dark, comfortable and secure.

Yet the parasite's total commitment to another species carries with it a certain insecurity. There is something vulnerable about an organism whose very existence depends on the health and future of another living species. Indeed, the parasite can be looked on as a sort of prisoner of the host, forced to accept host physiology and the rules of the house, rather than live as a free-roving individual. Moreover, it turns out to be a far from welcoming environment inside the host, whose body is nothing less than a living fortress, built to keep out foreigners. As soon as the parasite has gained entry, formidable defences come into action, and kill all but the experienced, well-adapted invader. Shortly after this first-line attack, a more ruthlessly efficient onslaught is unleashed, precisely targeted against the body of the foreigner. This is the attack of the immune system.

Surrounded by these hostile forces, which are described in Part 2, the parasite must not only stay alive but also, at the same time, reproduce itself, increase its numbers, and in the end leave the body of the host and be ready to enter new victims. To increase the likelihood of transfer large numbers of offspring must be formed, often of a specially heat- and drought-resistant variety (cysts, spores, worm eggs). A single human threadworm, for example, produces more than ten thousand eggs, which can survive in dust

---

Box 1 Parasites are tuned in to their chemical surroundings inside the host

Example 1 The virus of measles lives in the blood for about a week after it has infected a child, and from here it reaches the mucosa of the nose and throat where it multiplies, causing common cold-like symptoms. It then spreads to other individuals by coughs and sneezes, just like a common cold. It is a complete mystery how the virus going round in the blood knows that it has arrived in the nose and throat rather than in the kidney or muscles, but it obviously responds to delicate chemical cues.

Example 2 People living in parts of Africa, South America and Southeast Asia are liable to infection with a parasitic worm (*Wucheria bancrofti*) which is spread by mosquitoes and causes elephantiasis (gross enlargement, usually of the leg). The adult worm lives in the lymph channels of the groin and produces hundreds of microscopic larvae, each 1/100th of an inch long. These enter the blood and are picked up by mosquitoes for transfer to other people. The right mosquitoes, however, are night-biting mosquitoes, and the worm has adapted to this by liberating the larvae into the bloodstream only at night. Evidently the parasite responds to body changes taking place during each 24 hours (the so-called diurnal rhythm). Another parasitic worm (Loa loa, the eye worm in Africa) is spread by day-biting flies, and in this case the tiny larvae enter the blood only during daytime.

---

and under children's fingernails. Some parasites, such as those causing malaria and yellow fever, are fortunate enough to get free transport to the next host. They are taken up by mosquitoes, carried directly to the next host, and then injected under the skin.

So the parasite's life is not an easy one. Much of this book is a description of the body's amazing set of defences, and the enterprising methods used by microbial parasites to get round them.

We can summarize the parasite's problems as follows. If it is to be successful and survive as a species there are five obligatory steps it must take:

- It has to *attach to or enter* the host, surmounting the barriers and cleansing mechanisms present at the surfaces of the body, as described in Chapter 2.

- It must *evade the local defences* that are straightaway called into action and, if necessary, it must spread through the body.

- It must *multiply*, increasing its numbers or laying its eggs.

- It must *evade the powerful immune defences* (Chapter 3) for long enough to complete its business.

- Finally, because everything depends on this, the parasite must *leave the body* and spread to fresh hosts. To ensure this, it must make its exit from a suitable part of the body and in large enough numbers. The spread from one host to another is often so hazardous that very large numbers must be sent on the journey, and nearly all of them fall on stony ground and perish.

Nature needs balance, with limits to microbial damage

As we have already seen, causing disease is not a requirement. Too much damage to the host is unprofitable, because if the parasite regularly does this it will deplete the host species. A balance must be struck. Ideally the parasite should take what it needs, do what it has to do, and cause as little damage as possible. The common cold viruses, for instance, have got it right and are highly successful. After abundant multiplication in the nasal passages they stimulate a flow of virus-rich fluid from the nose, something which is needed for spread of the infection to the next person, but which causes no more than a day or two's discomfort.

For these reasons only a small proportion of the parasites infecting humans give rise to significant disease. Even those that have a bad reputation, such as polioviruses or meningococci, are harmless in most of us, multiplying and causing an asymptomatic infection so that they can be transmitted with minimum upset to other people. *Polioviruses* normally grow harmlessly in the intestine and are shed in the faeces to infect others. Unfortunately, in one or two infected persons per hundred, the virus invades the blood, reaches the brain, and causes a serious paralytic disease. This is what used to happen in the days before poliovaccines. And *meningococci*, which multiply in the nose and throat of many people without ill effect, very occasionally spread to the blood and invade the coverings of the brain to cause meningitis. The diseases (poliomyelitis, meningitis) that give these microbes their names are uncommon results of infection, and, from the point of view of the microbe, regrettable accidents because it is quite unnecessary for them to invade these parts of the body and injure the host.

13

The parasite versus the host

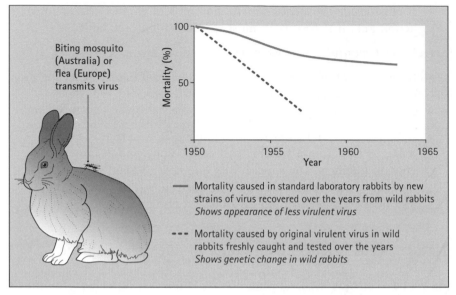

Figure 2 Myxomatosis in Australian rabbits.

Naturally enough the 'rogue' parasites such as HIV, rabies or anthrax, the ones that regularly cause damage and disease, are of great interest to physicians or veterinary surgeons. But you might ask why is it that such parasites are virulent rather than well-behaved. One reason is that they have not had time to become adapted to the host. This seems likely in the case of HIV, which has arrived quite recently in our species and has not yet settled down. Another reason is that the host in question is not actually necessary for the survival of the parasite, and this is true for rabies or psittacosis (parrot disease) in humans. The microbes responsible for these last two diseases have a life cycle that depends only on carnivorous animals (rabies) or birds (psittacosis). Humans are not needed, so it does not matter if they are damaged.

Myxomatosis in Australia

The best way to illustrate the sequence of events when the parasite causes too much damage to the host is to describe what happens when a highly virulent infectious agent is unleashed on a susceptible population. The story of myxomatosis in the Australian rabbit is the best-documented example, and it charts the origin and natural evolution of an infectious disease (Box 2).

Box 2 A plague on rabbits

Myxoma virus normally infects a certain species of rabbit that lives in South America (*Sylvilagus brasiliensis*). It is transmitted from rabbit to rabbit by mosquitoes, grows in the skin at the site of the mosquito bite, and causes a local swelling that acts as a rich source of virus from which other mosquitoes can be infected. It does not make the rabbit sick. Yet the same virus in the European species of rabbit (*Oryctolagus cuniculus*) causes a rapidly fatal disease. More than 90% of European rabbits die after infection.

Myxoma virus looked like the answer to the Australian farmer's prayer, the solution to the rabbit problem, and it was successfully introduced into the country in 1950. In the beginning, more than 99% of the rabbits died, but then, over the course of 5–10 years, two fundamental changes took place (Figure 2).

First, new and less lethal strains of virus appeared and replaced the original strain. This happened because rabbits infected with the less lethal strains survived longer, giving more time for the virus to be transmitted, and so these better-transmitted strains enjoyed a great advantage. Virulence was therefore lowered, although mortality did not reach zero because even in European rabbits a certain amount of spread, growth, and consequent damage by the virus was necessary to produce the virus-rich swellings on ears, nose and face, and ensure transmission.

The second change was that the rabbit population altered its character because those that were genetically more susceptible to the infection were eliminated, leaving the more resistant ones.

In other words, the less lethal types of virus proved to be more successful parasites because they were more readily transmitted. And the virus, by killing off genetically susceptible rabbits, selected out a more resistant population. If the rabbit population had been eliminated as was hoped, the virus also would have died out, but instead the host–parasite relationship settled down to a state of better balanced pathogenicity. Perhaps HIV in humans is destined to tread the same path.

Australian rabbits now face a new threat. This is a different virus (a calicivirus), which was introduced from Europe, and it spreads between rabbits by contact, causing a haemorrhagic disease. In contrast to myxomatosis, where a week or more's sickness is the rule, rabbits die within 24–48 hours, and for this reason the new virus is more acceptable to animal rights groups.

The parasite versus the host

The Sweating Sickness

This example is from humans, and although the story is similar it is less well charted. The *Sweating Sickness* was a dramatic disease that swept through England to cause five summer epidemics between 1485 and 1551. The sufferer developed headache, chest pain, severe sweating, and often died within 24 hours. As described by a contemporary physician in the florid language of that period '...it is on account of the fetid, corrupt, putrid and loathsome vapours close to the region of the heart and of the lungs whereby the panting of the breath magnifies and increases and restricts itself'. The disease seems to have come from Europe, the first epidemic beginning three weeks after the Earl of Richmond's army, which included mercenaries from France, entered London. It was no respecter of class or status, and the Lord Mayor of London, his successor, and six aldermen, all died within a week. The Sweating Sickness disappeared for good after 1551. It doesn't sound like any infectious disease that we know, so either it changed its nature and settled down as a less virulent, less recognizable infection, or else it burnt itself out and became extinct by exhausting the supply of uninfected susceptible people. The epidemics were so explosive that it was perhaps spread by coughs and sneezes, but it seems unlikely to have been influenza because this generally strikes in mid-winter.

When a damaging infectious disease first appears in one part of the world there is a weeding out of genetically susceptible people, so that the population becomes more resistant and the death rate is lowered, just as it did with myxomatosis in Australian rabbits. However, if the infection later spreads to other parts of the world, to islands or continents where there are previously unexposed and susceptible populations, it once again causes a much more serious disease. This is what happened with tuberculosis.

How tuberculosis has changed over the years

We know that susceptibility to tuberculosis depends a great deal on the genes, as was shown by a study on twins. Not everyone who is infected develops the disease, but if one of a pair of identical twins has the disease the other twin (with exactly the same genes) also had the disease in 98% of cases. In comparison, only 26% of non-identical twins were affected. During the great ravages of tuberculosis in European cities in the 17th to 19th centuries everyone became infected, just as they did with measles or mumps thirty years ago. Those whose genes made them susceptible to tuberculosis tended to be killed off, while the survivors passed on their resistance to their descendants. In this way tuberculosis brought about genetic changes in the population. As recently as 1850 more than 500 people in every 100,000 in

Boston, New York and European cities died of tuberculosis each year. Soon after this living conditions such as crowding and diet, which are also known to affect susceptibility to tuberculosis, slowly began to improve, and mortality began to fall. But when ships brought the infection to previously unexposed populations in Africa, Pacific Islands and other isolated places the effect was devastating. Among the Plains Indians in Saskatchewan, Canada, in 1886, the bacteria rapidly spread through the body of infected individuals to give a tuberculosis death rate of 9000 per 100,000. Just in case you are remembering what happened with myxomatosis in rabbits, we do not know whether the tuberculosis bacteria themselves have changed.

The iceberg effect
We have talked about disease and death after invasion by parasitic microbes. One of the messages is that it is uncommon for a parasite to cause exactly the same disease in all those that are infected. Both the severity and the exact clinical picture depend on variables such as age, sex, the genes, and the nutritional status of the host. Measles and cholera give a fairly regular type of disease, but others such as syphilis cause a wide range of symptoms and pathology.

Indeed, many infections can be without symptoms, which means that those showing signs of disease represent only the tip of the iceberg. The asymptomatically infected individuals become immune and resistant to reinfection, but during the infection they are not identified. They go about their normal affairs, stay in the community, and silently infect others.

PROBLEMS FOR THE HOST

Humans, like other species, have faced constant invasion by parasites. It has always been a fact of life. From the earliest stages of evolution, strong defences have been essential. When a new parasite comes into a species the effect can be devastating, as in the case of HIV in humans or myxomatosis in rabbits. Only those with good enough defences survived. An individual lucky enough to have genes that improved the defences is more likely to survive and hand on these genes to descendants.

The defences are of two types:

- Basic defences. The basic (early) defences include the wandering white cells whose job is to engulf (phagocytose) and destroy invaders, and the presence in body fluids of certain chemical weapons. These defences are ancient ones, present in all animals, and they come into action without delay.

17

- Immune defences. At a later stage in evolution another and more powerful type of defence system emerged. It was adaptive, in the sense that it was not switched on until the invader had been recognized as foreign, and it took at least a week to become effective. But it had the great advantage that it was 'tailor-made', specifically directed against the molecules of the invader. This was the *immune system*.

The power of the immune system is tremendous. People in whom it is not working (for instance those with depressed immunity due to HIV infection in AIDS) are killed by the parasites they would otherwise resist, or by resident microbes that are otherwise harmless. On the other hand, if the immune system 'runs amok' by attacking the host rather than (or as well as) the invader (so-called 'autoimmunity', see Box 5) it can cause life-threatening damage. Like that other powerful and potentially dangerous force, the blood clotting system, which is the body's defence against trauma, it needs to be carefully controlled.

Unfortunately *microbes multiply exceedingly rapidly* compared with their vertebrate hosts. The generation time of an average bacterium or virus is measured in hours, compared with about 20 years for the human host. Also the microbe's genetic equipment is much smaller, with less complicated controls, so that a minor change in the genes more easily leads to an important change in structure or behaviour. Bacteria, moreover, have the unique ability to hand over their genes (DNA) directly to other bacteria, even to unrelated bacteria. This happens when the genes, which are often genes causing resistance to antibiotics, are carried separately from the rest of the bacterial DNA, on structures called plasmids. The plasmid with its cargo of genes can pass directly across to the other bacterium. In this way advantageous genes present in one bacterium can rapidly be shared with quite different types of bacteria. In recent years staphylococci that acquired their resistance to antibiotics in this way and are a headache for physicians, have spread dramatically between different hospitals and different countries.

For these reasons microbes evolve with great speed in comparison with their hosts, and this means that they are generally many steps ahead of the host's defences, which are by no means infallible. If they were there would be no infectious diseases. If there are ways round the established defences, then some microbes are likely to have discovered and taken advantage of them. But the slowly evolving host has made its own response by improving and modifying the defences. The microbe, in turn, will respond with further adaptations, so that the picture is one of continual conflict, of changing strategies and counterstrategies. Also, because invaders will always exploit weak points, it has been unwise for the host to rely too much on a single method of defence. This is why, as we shall see, the defences often show duplication and overlap. In military terms there is a versatile, well-stocked armoury rather than just one or two good weapons.

Before we go into the nuts and bolts of the body's defences and talk about the ways in which microbes get round them, perhaps we should name the players in this ancient drama.

A ROGUE'S GALLERY OF MICROBIAL PARASITES OF HUMANS

Microbes are fairly recent arrivals on the medical scene. Diseases such as malaria, bubonic plague and smallpox have been known for hundreds of years, but it was not until good microscopes were invented in the 19th century that microbes became visible and were found to be guilty in so many diseases.

From a biological point of view the differences between the main groups of microbes are fundamental, breathtaking. So much so, that to describe a bacterium as a virus (a common practice in newspaper columns) is as inaccurate as describing a walrus as a type of grasshopper.

Size is another factor that is worth noting, as illustrated in Figure 3. When you consider a staphylococcus attempting to infect a person you have to picture an object a quarter of an inch high approaching Mount Everest, or an invisible speck measuring one five hundredth of an inch standing against St Paul's Cathedral, London. You can remove most microbes from a fluid by passing it through a porcelain filter. The ones that are not held back by the filter because they are small enough to get through ('filter-passing') are viruses.

Microbial *numbers* are almost as difficult to grasp. A single cough from a person with tuberculosis can discharge into the air 3000 bacteria, but breathing in just one of them may be enough to cause infection. Again, the stool of a child with viral diarrhoea may contain a thousand million viruses per gram, which is such a large number that an invisible faecal contamination of the hand will carry the infection. A cold sore can contain a million herpesviruses and a nose blow from a patient with lepromatous leprosy ten million leprosy bacteria. Figures such as these indicate that we are vastly outnumbered by our microbial parasites. If we count only the harmless resident bacteria described in Chapter 7, there are ten times as many of these as there are cells in the body. Strictly speaking we have always lived in the Age of Parasites. For comparison, it has been calculated that there are ten

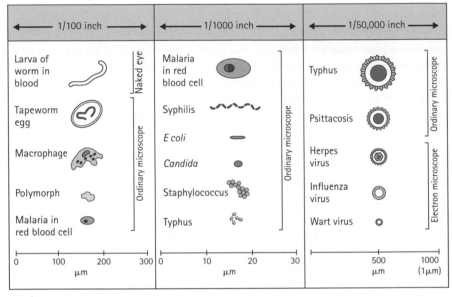

Figure 3 Too small to be seen — the size of microbes. Larva of worm in blood = *Wucheria bancrofti* (see Box 1). 25,000 staphylococci end to end = 1 inch. The (larval) worm shown is one of the smallest. The largest is 3 m long (tapeworm).

thousand million insects in the world for every human, but at least they are visible. Are we also living in the Age of Insects?

Here is the rogue's gallery

Prions – PRoteinaceous INfectious agents

These are puzzling microbes, the smallest, most primitive of all, whose nature is much discussed and argued about. They appear to contain neither DNA nor RNA and are thus different from viruses. Most scientists regard them as an abnormal form of a certain protein present in normal nerve cells and immune cells. Once the abnormal protein gets into a host cell it converts the normal into the abnormal form, and as the latter accumulates it eventually kills the cell. Prions (see Chapter 9) cause scrapie in sheep, BSE (bovine spongiform encephalopathy) in cattle, transmissible mink encephalopathy in mink, and in humans Creutzfeldt–Jakob disease (CJD), kuru, and fatal familial insomnia (FFI). Tiny holes appear in the brain, which takes on a spongy appearance, hence the name 'spongiform encephalopathy'.

Viruses

At least we understand these. They contain *either* DNA *or* RNA, packed in special capsules made of protein. The famous scientist and philosopher Sir Peter Medawar said that a virus is 'a piece of bad news wrapped in protein'. But it is not a cell, and on its own shows no signs of life. Multiplication takes place only inside living cells and then not simply by the virus dividing. This latter characteristic makes viruses fundamentally different from bacteria. The virus takes over the cell's metabolism, uses it as a factory to make more viruses, and after a day or so's intense biochemical activity hundreds of new viruses suddenly appear off the production line. DNA viruses include herpesviruses, adenoviruses and poxviruses, whereas RNA viruses include poliovirus, influenza, mumps, measles, rabies and yellow fever, etc. Unfortunately very few antiviral drugs are available, aciclovir and similar drugs for herpesviruses being the most successful ones. Viruses are ubiquitous, all-pervasive. Every species has its own collection. We will deal with the human ones, but there are thousands of others infecting bacteria, fungi, protozoa, plants, fish, insects, birds and mammals.

Bacteria

These microbes keep their genetic apparatus (DNA) in a single chromosome, which is not confined to a nucleus as in the case of the chromosomes of higher organisms. They also contain RNA. All multiply by cell division, and some of them only do so inside living host cells. Good antibacterial drugs are available (such as penicillin, cephalosporins) but antibiotic resistance is a growing problem. There are tens of thousands of different bacteria, and we can divide them into four groups.

Rickettsia	multiply only in living cells; cause diseases like Q fever, typhus, and Rocky Mountain spotted fever (the latter identified by Dr Howard T. Ricketts in 1906).
Chlamydia	multiply only in living cells, with a unique growth cycle; cause psittacosis, trachoma, urethritis.
Mycoplasma	differ from the others in having no cell wall; cause a type of pneumonia.
Regular bacteria	do not insist on living cells for multiplication, although some (e.g. tuberculosis) are capable of it. Cause gonorrhoea, tuberculosis, bacterial meningitis, typhoid, syphilis, etc.

Protozoa

Single-cell organisms; their DNA is separated from the rest of the cell and packaged into a nucleus, in several chromosomes. Multiply by cell division. Cause malaria, amoebic dysentery, trypanosomiasis, etc. Antiprotozoal drugs available (e.g. metronidazole).

Fungi

These too contain their DNA in several chromosomes. They can grow as single cells (like the moulds that grow on old bread and on shower curtains), in branching forms consisting of many cells (the fungi causing ringworm), or in either of these forms (*Candida*, causing thrush). Thick cell wall. Antifungal drugs available (nystatin, ketoconazole).

Worms (helminths)

A 3-metre-long tapeworm or a 30-centimetre-long roundworm (see Glossary) is hardly microbe-sized, but I am classing them as microbes for two reasons. First because their eggs and larvae (often used to diagnose infection) are microbe-sized. Second because as parasites they are subject to the same rules of engagement, confronted by the same host defences, and they employ the same parasite strategies as regular microbes. Worms, however, differ from regular microbes because of their complex structure, with nervous system and organs, and different developmental stages appropriate for their different hosts. They also differ because nearly all of them do not actually multiply (increase in numbers) in the vertebrate host. If you are infected with five worms the number stays at five. Eggs and larvae, however, are produced and dispatched in large numbers on their hazardous journey to new hosts.

Part 2

HOW WE DEFEND OURSELVES

'...thou hast set thine house of defence very high. There shall be no evil happen unto thee: nor shall any plague come nigh thy dwelling.'
                    Psalms 91, verse 9.

'The most vigorous individuals, or those which have most successfully struggled with their conditions of life, will generally leave most progeny. But success will often depend on having special weapons or means of defence, or on the charms of the males; and the slightest advantage will lead to victory.'
                    from *On the Origin of Species*
                    Charles Darwin (1809–1882)

Darwin was thinking about the struggle for existence in terms of competition for territory, food, females, or defence against predators. He died before the era of microbiology but his words apply equally well to defence against microbial invaders.

Our defences against microbial parasites operate at three levels, and the fact that there are these different levels makes sense from the point of view of military strategy, as illustrated in Figure 4.

- First, there are the *outer defences at the body surface*, the equivalent of the castle's moat and walls. They prevent the invader attaching to and entering the body in the first place.

- Second, should the microbe gain entry, there is a set of *early defences* that come into play almost immediately. They are the soldiers waiting behind the walls with their daggers and swords. All animals, from crabs and insects to frogs, birds and mammals, have these early defences and although they are primitive they are nevertheless powerful. Crabs and insects don't have an immune system but their early defences alone give them excellent protection.

- Third there are the *immune defences*, originally developed by primitive fish-like vertebrates, and which have been gradually upgraded during the evolution of warm-blooded birds and mammals. They are precisely targeted against each separate type of invader, are of immense power, and often decide the outcome. Perhaps we can compare them with the firearms that were added at a later date to the weapons of war – not replacing the earlier weapons and sometimes (e.g. the bayonet) joining forces with them.

Let us take a closer look at each of these defences.

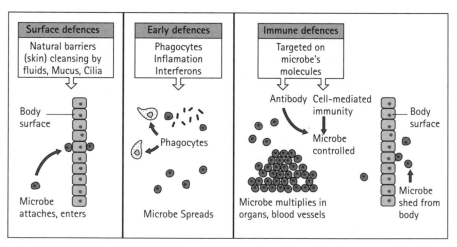

Figure 4 Our defences work at three levels.

Chapter 2

SURFACES BARRIERS AND
THE EARLY DEFENCES

'This animal is very bad; when attacked it defends itself'
from *La Menagerie*
(anon, French, 1868).

BODY SURFACES

If we greatly simplify the anatomy and forget details like muscles, brain, liver and heart, our body can be thought of as a *series of surfaces* that cover it and line its cavities, separating it off from the outside world (Figure 5). Each of the surfaces is lined by a carpet of specialized cells. They are the outer defences, walls of the host citadel, and with their local defensive devices, they form a wonderful protective barrier against invasion. Parasites have to gain a footing on either the outside or the inside of the body, and to do so must attach to or penetrate one of these surfaces. It is interesting to note that from this point of view parasites in the intestine, for instance, although in one sense inside the body, are still really at the body surface and have not penetrated any deeper than this.

Skin

The external surface is covered by *skin*, a dry, horny, material. It consists of many layers of cells, the outermost of which are dead. With its strength and elasticity skin gives good mechanical protection, especially when covered with hair, and incidentally it is one of the biggest immune

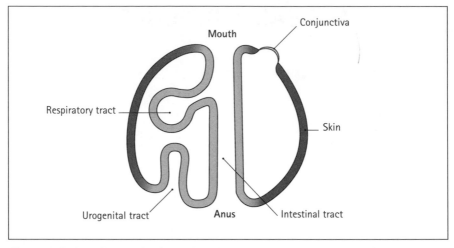

Figure 5 Body surfaces as barriers to invasion.

strongholds in the body. At the skin surface it is slightly acid, which is unfavourable for many microbes, and the very dryness of most parts of the skin makes it a hostile environment. If you moisten an area of skin by covering it with a polythene sheet there is a large increase in the number of bacteria. Invasion through the skin generally follows a local injury or a bite (a small bite from a mosquito, a larger one from a dog), but there are one or two parasites that can burrow through on their own, such as the bacteria of leptospirosis or the parasitic worm causing schistosomiasis (see Glossary).

If only the defences at all body surfaces could be as strong as those at the skin! Unfortunately in other parts of the body we are forced to allow more intimate contact and exchange with the outside world. Thus, where food is absorbed (the intestines), gases exchanged (the lungs), and urine and sexual products discharged (the urinary and genital channels), the lining consists of no more than a few layers of cells, and these cells are alive. In the eye the thick skin is replaced by a transparent layer of living cells, the conjunctiva. All these surfaces are very vulnerable, offering attractive opportunities to invaders, and each is therefore provided with automatic cleansing mechanisms and local defence systems. To be successful a microbial parasite must be able to circumvent them (Figure 6).

Conjunctiva
The *conjunctiva* is kept moist and healthy by the continuous flow of

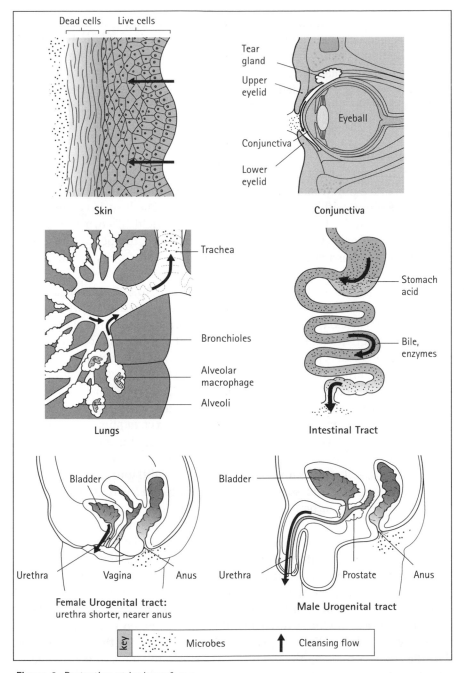

Figure 6 Protection at body surfaces.

secretions from local glands. Every few seconds there is the firm but gentle windscreen wiper action of the eyelids. The secretions themselves (tears) contain antimicrobial substances such as lysozyme, which destroys many bacteria, but their main action is a mechanical one, washing away foreign materials. Microbes approaching this part of the body have a chance only if they can stick onto the conjunctiva, or when there is something wrong with the cleansing system.

Respiratory tract

In the *nasal cavity and the lungs* special cells secrete mucus, which covers the surface as a thin film. Fine hairs (cilia) projecting from other cells move the mucus along with a regular to and fro beat. The beat is co-ordinated and from above looks like the movement of a field of corn in a gentle breeze. Inhaled particles, whether living or dead, are trapped in the mucus sheet, and then carried by ciliary action (up from the lungs or backwards from the nose) to the throat, where they are swallowed. The whole thing functions as a 'mucociliary escalator', and about 10,000 microbes a day, nearly all of them harmless, are inhaled in the air and dealt with in this way. Large particles, whether watery droplets or specks of dust, land in the nasal passages. The smallest particles of all, of the size that could contain a single tuberculosis bacterium or a virus, can go right down into the lungs and reach its terminal chambers, the alveoli, where they are engulfed by the phagocytes that lie in wait here (Figure 6). The largest particles or irritating materials are expelled with a hurricane blast of air (sneeze or cough). Many respiratory microbes, by the way, have learnt to stimulate sneezing or coughing, and thus ensure their successful dispersal from the body after multiplying in the nasal cavity and lungs.

It follows that if an invading microbe is to avoid the usual fate of a foreign particle it must do something to avoid being carried away by the mucociliary system or being killed by the phagocytes.

Intestinal tract

In the *mouth*, the flushing action of saliva provides a natural cleansing mechanism. Each day, about a litre is secreted, needing 400 swallows. As on most of the other body surfaces (see Part 4) there are large numbers of harmless resident bacteria (tens of millions per drop of saliva) specially adapted to life in this region. Their number is increased four-fold between meals, when salivary flow is greatly reduced and allows them to accumulate. Parasites colonizing the mouth must be able to attach to teeth, tongue, cheek or throat, or they will be rinsed away by saliva and swallowed.

The cleansing mechanism in the *intestine* is the steady downward flow of the contents. Diarrhoea and vomiting can be considered as giving extra, emergency, flushing action. To establish themselves here parasites must avoid being borne along in the dark, often hostile stream, and thrown out in the faeces. They will have to run the gauntlet of stomach acid, bile and digestive enzymes, which are damaging to many of them, and it is not easy to make close contact with the living cells lining the intestine because they are blanketed with a viscous layer of mucus. The deterrent action of acid is illustrated by the fact that if you give a human volunteer a drink that contains cholera or typhoid bacteria, the number of bacteria needed to cause infection is reduced at least a hundred-fold if the volunteer takes some bicarbonate of soda at the same time, to neutralize stomach acid.

The infant's intestine is notoriously vulnerable to infection, partly because it contains much less acid and partly because its immune defences are less well developed. This is why breast milk is such a valuable maternal gift, containing antibodies and other protective substances.

Urogenital tract

The main method for cleansing the *urinary and genital channels* and keeping out intruders is the downward flow of urine. Under normal circumstances the bladder is sterile, and the first task for a microbe invading the urethra (Figure 6) is to avoid being rinsed out during urination. If it does manage to reach the bladder it will escape being washed out if it can stick to the bladder wall, or if bladder emptying is incomplete and leaves behind a residual 'sump' of urine in which it can multiply. There are differences between the sexes. In the male, urinary infections (bladder infections or cystitis) are uncommon and are seen when something goes wrong with the flushing action of urine. Thus, an elderly man with an enlarged prostate gland suffers urinary infections because the enlarged gland surrounds the urethra and throttles it, so that the bladder cannot be completely emptied.

Things are more complicated in females because anatomy takes a hand and makes them very vulnerable. Not only is the urethra shorter (5 cm as opposed to 20 cm in the male), which means that bacteria have a shorter journey up into the bladder to cause cystitis, but it also suffers from a perilous proximity to the anus, which is a constant source of intestinal bacteria. Hence urinary infections are about 14 times commoner in women. The vagina, moreover, is subject to repeated introduction of a foreign object (the penis) which sometimes bears disease-producing microbes. Nature has responded to this threat of infection by providing additional local defences. During reproductive life the lining of the vagina contains glycogen, and the particular bacteria (lactobacilli, similar to the ones in yoghurt) that colonize the normal vagina make use of the glycogen and in doing so produce lactic acid. As a result, the vagina is slightly acid (pH about 5.0, see Glossary) and because most microbes are damaged by acid this discourages colonization by all but the lactobacilli themselves and a few other harmless bacteria. Microbes have the opportunity to invade when the defences are interfered with by objects, such as tampons, or when in older women there is a shortage of glycogen in the vagina due to a fall in oestrogen production. They are also helped when they have their own method for attaching to the cells lining the vagina or cervix.

Let us now examine what I have called the early defences, the ones that are ready for instant action. They work in three ways. First by switching on *inflammation*, second by letting the *phagocytes* do their deadly work, and third by mobilizing *chemical weapons* such as the interferons and complement.

INFLAMMATION – IT FEELS BAD BUT IS A WONDERFUL DEVICE

Inflammation is what happens when a finger, toe, or any part of the body becomes red, swollen and painful. It is due to changes in small blood vessels. In a normal, uninfected part of the body these small blood vessels bring oxygen, glucose and other nutrients to the cells and take away carbon dioxide and waste products. It is a two-way traffic, and the materials exchanged are all small molecules.

Occasionally larger (protein) molecules leave the small blood vessels and enter tissues, and so do a few white blood cells called lymphocytes (see Glossary). The proteins and cells are not returned directly to the blood, but first enter tiny channels called lymphatics (Figure 7). These channels, containing a colourless fluid called lymph, connect up to local lymph stations (nodes). After passing through the node the lymph runs into larger channels and eventually reaches the blood. All this takes place under normal conditions, especially at the body surfaces, and is on a small scale. But as soon as a microbial invader has entered, the body reacts locally with a tremendous increase in the 'leakage' of proteins and white blood cells from small blood vessels. This is what lies behind inflammation, and it is the body's method for rushing protective antibodies (proteins) and white cells to the site of infection. The blood vessels are the supply lines that bring the soldiers and ammunition to the battlefield. Things move quickly once the microbe has breached the body surface and has begun to spread and mul-

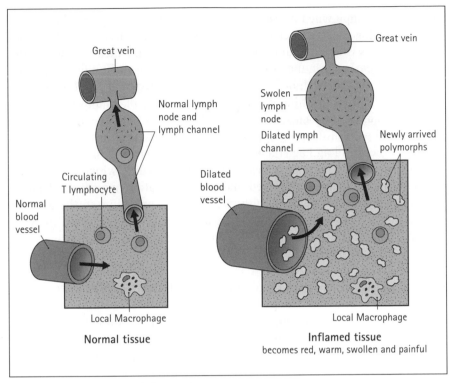

Figure 7 What happens in inflammation.

tiply. Speed is essential, and a few hours' delay on the part of the host can be disastrous. Inflammation therefore begins with a *dramatic dilation of small blood vessels*, which allows a protein-rich fluid containing antibodies (and complement, see below) to seep through the blood vessel wall and into the tissues. In addition, white cells in the blood stick to the walls of the inflamed vessels and then move rapidly through them and out into tissues. Moderate numbers of phagocytic cells (the residents) are already there, but much larger numbers (especially those called polymorphs, see below) now pour in from the blood. The affected area, because of the dilated blood vessels, becomes **red** and **warm** and is **swollen** by the fluid and cells that are passing into it (Figure 7). It feels **painful**. Lymphatic channels are also dilated, and the flow of lymph increases as the fluid, containing the white cells and microbes, is drained away.

The white cells (phagocytes and immune cells) are already locked in the battle with the invader. Any free microbes and many of the cells are filtered

31

off from the lymph when it reaches the node. Lymph nodes are military out-posts of the host defence network, because as well as filtering off microbes they are places where immune responses are started. By focusing everything into these nearby immune strongholds the body can often deal with the infection at a local level, before it has a chance to spread any further.

Suppose a cut on your hand gets contaminated with an unpleasant bac-terium such as a streptococcus. The next day the cut has become red, warm, swollen and painful. The tiny lymph channels in the skin form a dense net-work and the invading bacteria will have entered them within minutes. They are carried up to the lymph nodes in the armpit (axilla), which enlarge and feel sore, and sometimes a fine red line of inflammation appears up the arm, marking the position of the lymph channel as it passes up to the axillary lymph node. Your defences have been mobilized, which is good for you, and in a few days' time the infection will be overcome.

In the old days before antibiotics, a boil in the skin was often treated with a hot poultice. The word poultice dates from the 16th century, and consisted of a soft paste spread onto a piece of muslin or linen, which was heated and then applied to the boil. The paste held the heat and it acted by increasing the amount of inflammation, a worthy aim because it brought extra sup-plies of phagocytes and antibodies to the infected area.

In recent years scientists have sorted out the complex chemical events that take place during inflammation, and have discovered that a great assortment of molecules are responsible. Supposing we ask how a white cell suspended in the blood flowing through a small blood vessel knows that the region it is passing through is inflamed. Apparently it recognizes a spe-cial type of molecule called a *selectin* that has now appeared on the surface of the cells lining the local blood vessels. Instead of passing by the white cell sticks to this molecule, and then it migrates through the vessel wall and into tissues. If the selectin molecule is not displayed inflammation is min-imal, white blood cells are not delivered, invading bacteria are not dealt with, and the individual suffers chronic skin infections. You can also demonstrate the importance of inflammation by injecting adrenalin under the skin. This shuts off local blood vessels and prevents the inflammatory response. Local invaders will now multiply more readily and cause a more severe infection.

But too much inflammation is bad for you. Inflammation, although locally so beneficial, could be harmful for the body as a whole if it took place on a very large scale, or if it took place simultaneously in many dif-ferent parts of the body. It would lead to widespread opening up of small blood vessels, and enough plasma (the fluid part of blood) would leak out into the tissues to cause collapse of the circulation and shock, just as if there had been a massive haemorrhage. There is therefore a special control system to prevent inflammation becoming too widespread. It is centred in the brain and adrenal gland, and acts by releasing *steroid hormones* to damp down the inflammatory response. This is why certain diseases caused by inflammation, such as rheumatoid arthritis, are treated by giving the patient steroid hormones.

THE PHAGOCYTES, ESSENTIAL WEAPONS IN THE EARLY DEFENCES

George Bernard Shaw (1856–1950) was convinced of their usefulness!
'There is at bottom only one genuinely scientific treatment for all diseases, and that is to stimulate the phagocytes.'
From The Doctor's Dilemma (1911).

The Russian zoologist *Elie Metchnikov* was born in 1845. After various misfortunes and two attempts at suicide (once with an overdose of morphia and once by inoculating himself with blood from a patient suffering from relapsing fever (see Glossary), following which he developed the disease but recovered), Metchnikov settled in Messina, Italy, and at the marine biology laboratory carried out his famous studies on sea anenomes and starfish.

Under the microscope he had seen certain mobile cells in starfish larvae, and one day in 1882, in his own words:

'...a sudden thought flashed across my brain. It struck me that similar cells might serve in the defence of the organism against intruders. Feeling that there was something in this of surpassing interest, I felt so excited that I began striding up and down the room and even went to the seashore to collect my thoughts. I said to myself that, if my supposition was true, a splinter introduced into the body of a starfish larva, devoid of blood vessels or of a nervous system, should soon be surrounded by mobile cells as is to be observed in the man who runs a splinter into his finger. This was no sooner said than done...'

He introduced a rose thorn under the skin of one of the starfish larvae, and the next morning ('I had been too excited to sleep that night') he examined the larva under the microscope. He was able to see, through the larva's transparent skin, that the thorn had been surrounded by mobile cells. The same cells would engulf particles of carmine dye.

From this and later observations on mammalian white blood cells (leucocytes) in Louis Pasteur's laboratory in Paris, Metchnikov became convinced that such cells (he called them *phagocytes*) were important in resistance to bacterial and other infections. Incidentally, like many famous scientists, he had his blind spots. He did not believe that substances in the serum (the antibodies we now know to be crucial!) had anything to do with phagocytosis, insisting that they were only products of disintegrating phagocytes!

Metchnikov described two types of phagocyte, large ones he called *macrophages* ('large eaters'), and small ones with a lobed nucleus called microphages ('small eaters'), now known as polymorphonuclear leucocytes or *polymorphs*. Both are present in the blood and they are white cells, as opposed to the red cells that make blood red.

The other type of white blood cell is the lymphocyte, a small immune cell that is not a phagocyte. We can therefore divide white blood cells into:

- *polymorphs* and *macrophages* (the two types of phagocyte);

- *lymphocytes* (which are the subject of Chapter 4).

Phagocytes are ready for instant action against invading microbes. You are looking down a microscope at a phagocyte, one of thousands present in a drop of blood you obtained from a pricked finger. It is in a salty solution in a warm glass chamber and has settled down onto the glass. Although it has begun to move around it is nevertheless attached to the glass and can't easily be rinsed off. You now add a very small amount of baker's yeast to the fluid, and as the tiny yeast cells come tumbling down round the phagocyte the action begins. Since it landed on the glass of the culture chamber the phagocyte has been moving, sending out processes in all directions as if exploring the surrounding territory. Soon one of these processes comes into contact with a yeast cell. It sticks to the yeast cell. Now, if you watch patiently for a few more minutes, you will see the phagocyte forming a sort of cup round its victim, flowing round it and eventually completely enclosing it. As the package or vacuole containing the trapped yeast cell sinks inside the phagocyte the prisoner gradually begins to look fuzzy, then it disintegrates, and finally disappears. The yeast cell has been phagocytosed, killed and digested, with much the same sequence of events as when a free-living amoeba takes up and digests its microscopic prey.

Let us consider these events in more detail, and see how they relate to what actually happens in the body. Whether the phagocytes are local ones lying in readiness under the skin, or whether the inflammatory response has just called them out from small blood vessels in the vicinity (Figure 8), they will have to move about if they are to carry out their attack on an invader. They cannot be expected to congregate at the exact site without any guidance. Guidance is given by substances formed around the invading bacteria by complement (see Glossary), and also by substances released by the bacteria themselves. The phagocytes sense these substances, migrate to their source, and thus assemble in the right place. The process is called *chemotaxis* (movement to chemicals). Once they are on site phagocytosis can begin, and scientists have now dissected out the events in terms of the actual molecules concerned.

The chamber engulfing the prisoner is called the phagocytic vacuole and is the cell's stomach. Generally things proceed smoothly, but sometimes there is regurgitation of food, indigestion, or the cell can suffer from food- poisoning.

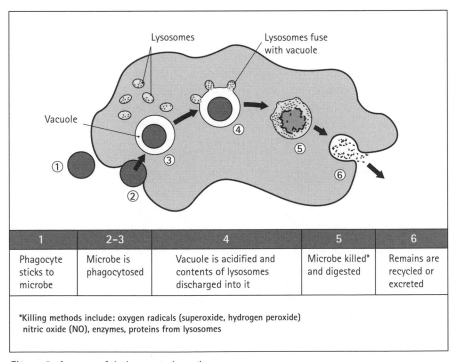

1	2–3	4	5	6
Phagocyte sticks to microbe	Microbe is phagocytosed	Vacuole is acidified and contents of lysosomes discharged into it	Microbe killed* and digested	Remains are recycled or excreted

*Killing methods include: oxygen radicals (superoxide, hydrogen peroxide) nitric oxide (NO), enzymes, proteins from lysosomes

Figure 8 A successful phagocyte in action.

How phagocytes work

The chemical basis for the phagocyte recognizing and sticking to the foreign invader is still something of a mystery when it takes place early in the infection. Later, recognition is enormously enhanced by the antibodies that have been formed against the microbe and which attach to it, acting as opsonins, as described below.

As soon as the phagocyte has stuck to the microbe a series of events are triggered off in the cell. Supposing a polymorph phagocyte meets and attaches to *Escherichia coli*, the resident bacterium of the intestine. A successful outcome, for the host that is, can be outlined as follows.

- The cell begins to engulf the microbe and this needs energy, which is provided by oxidizing (burning) glucose, so that the respiration rate in the cell increases 10–20 times. The necessary physical movements during the embracing and engulfing of the victim (stages 2 and 3 in Figure 8) are carried out by the cell's own muscles (known as actin and myosin filaments) which are anchored to a skeleton (microtubules) in the cytoplasm. The microbe is soon completely enclosed in a vacuole.

- It now becomes *acid* in the vacuole, the pH falling to 5.0 or lower, and this in itself damages many microbes. Next, a group of harmless-looking little sacs (called 'granules' or *lysosomes*) present in the phagocyte start to move towards the vacuole. They contain a formidable battery of chemical weapons, which are poured onto the captured microbe as the sacs fuse with the vacuole (stage 4 in Figure 8). These antimicrobial weapons would also damage the phagocyte, so naturally they have to be kept in special sacs.

- What takes place now is a miracle of molecular ingenuity, and after a few minutes' exposure to this sacful of enzymes and other substances the microbe is dead. However, immediately after they have been killed the bacteria seem still to be intact and it is not until another 15–30 minutes that they look moth-eaten and start to disintegrate. Complete digestion and disposal of the corpse can take a lot longer.

When we say the microbe is dead we mean that it can no longer divide and multiply when freed from the phagocyte. In the case of *E. coli* we can check for this in the laboratory by spreading the bacteria on the surface of a suitably nutritious jelly-like material, placing the container overnight in an incubator at blood temperature, and seeing whether visible heaps (colonies) of bacteria have been formed next morning. If none are present it means there has been no multiplication of bacteria, and we say they are dead. This is why the word *sterile* (= devoid of offspring) comes to be used. Of course, one has to be careful. We may not have provided ideal conditions for bacterial growth, or the bacteria may be very slow growing, or they may be there, still alive in the usual sense, waiting for a better opportunity to multiply. And very different methods of testing are needed for viruses or other microbes that grow only in living cells.

Although the phagocyte needed oxygen to manufacture much of the antimicrobial cocktail delivered to the vacuole, especially the powerful items called oxygen radicals (see Glossary), it can kill without it. Phagocytes often have to do their work in parts of the body where the oxygen supply is poor, such as in damaged or dying tissues, and it is here that many bacteria (the ones called anaerobes = without air) actually prefer to multiply. Hence the phagocyte has additional weapons that do not depend on an oxygen supply.

I have told the story for the polymorph type of phagocyte. If we went into more detail we would see that macrophages have a slightly different set of antimicrobial weapons, which means that the two types of phagocyte differ in the speed and efficiency with which they deal with microbes.

This is the time to mention pus. Pus is a well-known product of infection and inflammation. The stuff of boils and abscesses. It contains bacteria, both dead and alive, and phagocytes, and the fluid debris from the battlefield. Pus can be thick and milky (from staphylococcal infection), blood-stained and watery (streptococci), cheesy (tuberculosis), or foul-smelling (anaerobic bacteria). It is a less common sight in these days of antibiotics and hygiene, but it at least means that the phagocytes are there and doing their best. In the old days it was referred to as 'laudable' (praiseworthy) pus (see Box 21).

More about the life of phagocytes

Macrophages

Richard had himself tattooed when he was 18. Nothing special, just a coiled serpent with stars round it on his forearm, and coloured bright blue and deep red. He was pleased with the result, and liked the details of the serpent's teeth and the flames leaping out of its mouth. But now, 25 years later, the outline has become less clear, it looks blacker, and the serpent has a fuzzy edge. It no longer has that clean fresh look.

What has happened is perfectly normal, and it tells us something about the habits and life span of *macrophages*. When the tattooist injected those pigments into Richard's skin the local phagocytes, which were macrophages, did their job and took up (phagocytosed) the pigment. A few of them found their way up to the lymph nodes in his armpit. But the pigments proved to be indigestible, and most of the cells stayed put in the skin, immobilized by their burden, still full of the bright colours. The artistic outline on Richard's forearm was retained. It was not for several months that the first macrophages began to age and die. Fresh young macrophages now came and engulfed the remains, and this continued over the years. During the repeated cycles of cell death followed by reuptake of the debris the macrophages with their load of pigment had moved around a bit in the skin, and this is why the outline of the serpent eventually became fuzzy. It looked blacker because the black pigment (Indian ink) was the most indigestible, the hardest to clear away.

Macrophages are not only long-lived (months or years) but they can undergo dramatic increases in antimicrobial powers when required. They work in close partnership with immune cells and with antibody, and have great ability to adapt their response according to the circumstances. Some of them circulate in the blood, having been formed in the bone marrow. These are in a resting state, but after leaving the blood and entering a site of infection they respond by forming dozens of different antimicrobial substances, becoming 'activated'.

Other macrophages are stationed more permanently at strategic sites in the body, in places (Figure 9) where they are likely to meet invading microbes. For instance they lie in wait under the surface of the skin, the intestine and the respiratory tract. Others monitor the lymph as it passes through the lymph nodes on its way back to the blood from the tissues. Others monitor the blood itself, lining the walls of special small blood vessels in the liver and spleen. Finally there are those that keep watch in the so-called 'body cavities'. The lungs and intestines are covered with a protective sheet of cells and an adjacent sheet of cells lines the wall of the chest and abdomen. The two sheets slide smoothly over each other during the movements of breathing and digestion. In between the two cell sheets are what we call the pleural and peritoneal 'cavities', although they are only potential cavities. They are dangerous places, vulnerable to microbial invasion if there is damage to the lungs or intestines. As if in expectation of such events, the cavities are lined by a rich collection of macrophages

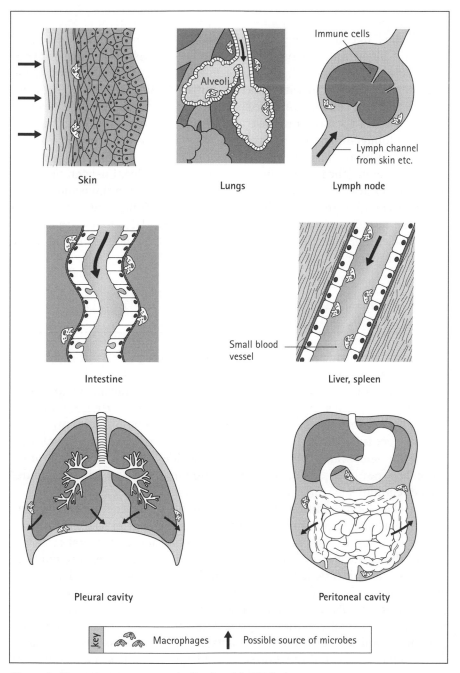

Skin

Lungs

Immune cells

Alveoli

Lymph node

Lymph channel from skin etc.

Intestine

Small blood vessel

Liver, spleen

Pleural cavity

Peritoneal cavity

key Macrophages ↑ Possible source of microbes

Figure 9 Macrophages are strategically placed in the body.

Polymorphs

Polymorphs, like macrophages, are formed in the bone marrow and circulate in the blood, only leaving it in places where there is inflammation. They are smaller, more compact, and faster moving cells, fully equipped at the time of their formation with amazing antimicrobial weaponry. They are ready for instant action, do-or-die soldiers, ready to discharge their weapons but unable to adjust the response according to the circumstances, unable to take a longer-term view like the macrophages. They live only for a day, either dying on the battlefield, or, if not given the opportunity to use their weapons, being called back from the blood and recycled. Co-operation with antibody is a feature of their action. A total of about ten thousand million (10^{10}) polymorphs are present in blood; and 10^{11} old ones are removed and the same number of new ones produced each day! To cope with sudden emergencies a massive reserve supply of 3×10^{12} polymorphs is held in the bone marrow, their total weight being about 100 grams.

CHEMICAL WEAPONS; INTERFERONS AND OTHER SUBSTANCES IN EARLY DEFENCE

This is the time to mention complement, interferons and cytokines. The phagocytes in Metchnikov's starfish larva must have been able to recognize foreign objects without the help of antibodies because starfish do not have antibodies. Antibodies are formed only in vertebrate animals with a proper immune system. A more primitive type of recognition was always necessary during the hundreds of millions of years of evolution before the appearance of vertebrates. How does this sort of recognition work, how does the phagocyte sense foreign material and what molecules are concerned?

More than a dozen different molecules are involved, and the *complement system* plays an important part (Box 7). Complement reacts with certain molecules, such as the endotoxins and the polysaccharides that are present on the surface of viruses, bacteria, and other microbes. The complement system is thus switched on. Some of its molecules cause inflammation as described earlier, and others are deposited on the surface of the microbe. Phagocytes are able to recognize these complement components and attach to them, thus literally getting to grips with the microbe. This is what triggers off phagocytosis. Complement acts as an opsonin, as described more fully on pages 60–61. As will be seen in Chapter 4, complement also helps in the working of the immune system. Indeed it can be thought of as a sort of link between more primitive ('natural') defences and the sophisticated immune defences.

The *cytokines* are molecules by which cells communicate with each other during immune responses. They are the hormones of the immune system. More than 40 different ones have been discovered, some coming into play early, when an immune response is just starting up, and others at a later stage. Altogether they form a complicated network of molecules which gives co-ordinated control over the mobilization, stimulation, and the switching off of immune cells. Important cytokines are the various interleukins (so far 18 different ones!), tumour necrosis factor and the interferons (alpha, beta and gamma).

I mention cytokines here because a few of them can be formed independently of immune responses and thus have a part to play in early defence. Interleukin-1 and tumour necrosis factor are released from macrophages at a very early stage in an infection, and after entering the blood they have widespread effects on the host. They get the body as a whole ready for the emergency by making the liver produce a special set of protective substances, and they also raise the body temperature.

Interleukin-1 formed in macrophages is the one that raises the body temperature to cause *fever*, especially at a later stage when the immune response comes into action. It sets the thermostat in the brain at a higher level, and in addition breaks down muscle proteins to yield emergency energy supplies for the coming struggle. Interferons as well as interleukin-1 are released into the blood and these substances are what cause many of the subjective feelings of illness. The infected individual, blissfully ignorant of this flurry of defence activity taking place inside him, begins to feel unwell and develops headache and muscle aches with the fever.

Fever is such a regular feature of infection, so unpleasantly associated with feeling unwell and having aches and pains that we think of it as a disadvantage. But a higher body temperature means increased metabolic activity in cells, which means faster and better responses in immune cells and phagocytes. Immune responses are undoubtedly increased. In the 17th century the English physician Thomas Sydenham wrote that 'Fever is a mighty engine which Nature brings into the world for the conquest of her enemies.' Indeed, in two infections, gonorrhoea and syphilis, the microbes are actually killed at febrile temperatures. It is curious that fever is not a notable feature in these particular diseases, and in the old days before antibiotics, patients were treated by injection with malaria parasites. This caused a good fever, enough to eradicate the gonorrhoea or syphilis, and afterwards they were given quinine to cure the malaria! This was such an important addition to the physician's meagre armoury that in 1927 Julian Wagner Jauregg, an Austrian neurologist and pioneer in this type of fever treatment, was awarded the Nobel Prize in Physiology and Medicine. At Horton Hospital in England, between 1922 and 1950, more than 10,000 people suffering from syphilis were treated with malaria.

Professor Ludwig Traube introduced the clinical thermometer into his hospital wards in Berlin in 1850. It was nine inches long, was used in the axilla (he considered the mouth and fist unreliable and the rectum indecent), and took 20 minutes to register. Fevers above 41°C can cause damage to cells, but even children, who easily run high temperatures, rarely exceed 40°C, a temperature commonly found in marathon runners after the race.

People still argue about how useful fever is in host defence because the actual evidence for other infections is not overwhelming. But it costs a great deal of energy to raise the body temperature and it is such an ancient and regular response that it must surely do more good than harm. Next time we reach for a drug like aspirin to bring the temperature down we should remind ourselves that fever, perhaps, is more than a regrettable by-product of infection – it is one of nature's ways of dealing with it.

Interferons are so-called because they interfere with the growth of viruses in host cells. In 1957 two virologists working in laboratories in Mill Hill, London, A. Isaacs and J. Lindemann, had been puzzled because a culture of living cells infected with one virus was often resistant to infection with another quite different virus. They thought that something might be released from infected cells that made the remaining cells insusceptible to the second virus. So they removed fluid from the cell cultures after the first virus infection and added the fluid to a new batch of cells. The new set of cells were now protected from the second virus. The scientists called the material responsible 'interferon', and later the actual molecules were isolated and characterized. We now know that there are three types of interferon (alpha, beta and gamma), and interferons alpha and beta are released from cells very early, only a few hours after they have been infected by a virus. They are important in early defence because they are formed by the first cells in the body to be infected, whether skin cells, intestinal cells, brain cells or liver cells. The interferons attach to nearby uninfected cells, making them resistant to a multitude of other viruses, and the effect lasts for a day or so. The message is that most viruses stimulate cells to produce interferons, and the interferons then act against most viruses.

Chapter 3

IMMUNE DEFENCES

*'I have made this letter longer than usual only because
I have not had the time to make it shorter.'*
From *Lettres Provincales*
Blaise Pascal (1623–1662).

The following is perhaps the hardest part of the book, and you can short-cut it by turning to the summaries at the end of this section (pages 68–69). It sets out the basic facts about immunity and how it works for our benefit. It is the nuts and bolts of the subject, and the story is not always simple because nature is not always simple. But if you grasp the basics you will then have a good understanding of what happens in your body during an infectious disease, how the formidable immune defences do their life-saving work, and how vaccines work for the benefit of mankind. You will also learn something about the wisdom of the body, and appreciate that beneficial responses can at the same time be harmful. The immune weapon is a two-edged sword, it needs to be kept under control, and the best strategy for the body is often one of compromise.

A ROYAL EXPERIMENT AND THE BEGINNINGS OF IMMUNOLOGY

Smallpox was no respecter of royalty, as illustrated by the story of Anne (1665–1725), Queen of Great Britain and Ireland, who contracted the disease when she was 12 years old. As the wife of Prince George of Denmark she became pregnant no less than 17 times, and all but one of the children were stillborn or died in infancy. Three of them died of smallpox, including the one that had survived infancy.

During the 1721 smallpox epidemic in England the youngest child of the Prince and Princess of Wales (Caroline of Ansbach) fell ill and it was at first thought to be the dreaded smallpox. It was not, but the Princess took notice when Lady Mary Wortley Montague, wife of the British Ambassador to Turkey, returned to England and sang the praises of a method of inoculation against smallpox. Lady Montague had had her six-year-old son inoculated. The technique was to take material from a skin lesion on a smallpox sufferer and inoculate it into the skin of the person to be protected. This caused an illness (not so bad as true smallpox that killed one in five of those who got it), and the person was now protected. The Turks (into the skin) and the Chinese (into the nostril) had been doing it for many years.

A group of physicians, reluctant to risk the procedure on a royal child, asked the King (George 1) if they could first try it out on condemned criminals in Newgate Prison, who would subsequently be pardoned. Permission was granted, and on August 9, 1721, three male and three female prisoners were inoculated, in the presence of 25 eminent physicians, surgeons and apothecaries. Each prisoner developed a brief illness (except one who turned out to have had smallpox already), and all were pardoned. One of them, a 19-year-old woman, was then ordered to 'lie every Night in the Same Bed (with a ten-year-old smallpox victim) and to attend to him constantly from the first Beginning of the Distemper to the very end'. She remained well. Then six more adults were successfully inoculated, and finally, to make quite sure, five orphans in St James Parish, Westminster.

The numbers were ridiculously small by today's standards, and only one individual had been tested for actual resistance to smallpox. Nevertheless, the physicians (and the newspapers) were now satisfied that it was safe enough, and on April 11, 1722, the 11-year-old Princess Amelia and the nine-year-old Princess Caroline were successfully inoculated.

But this type of inoculation never became very popular. For one thing it was not without hazards. and could make you very ill. In the following year 897 people were inoculated in the British Isles, America and Hanover, and 17 of them died. The method was eventually outlawed by an Act of Parliament in 1840. It was not until 1798 that the next big step against smallpox was taken, by Edward Jenner (see pages 155–156). In his original work he inoculated cowpox into seven people, but only two of them were subsequently tested for resistance to smallpox.

The first to carry out a scientifically designed experiment in immunology was Louis Pasteur, when in 1880 he inoculated groups of chickens with attenuated (weakened) chicken cholera bacteria, and showed that the birds were then protected against the lethal disease.

Neither Jenner nor Pasteur understood exactly how their inoculations had made the people or the chickens immune, but the science of immunology had been inaugurated. And in the late 20th century we are still dotting the Is and crossing the Ts!

THE IMMUNE SYSTEM

The immune system, like the history of the world, can be set out on the back of a postcard or in several heavy volumes, and this account is something in between. We will begin at the beginning.

For thousands of millions of years the basic cleaning and early defence systems outlined in the last chapter, sometimes called *natural immunity*, have been the mainstay of defence. But they are always the same, not modified by experience, and perhaps rather sluggish for warm-blooded vertebrates. Something more adaptable, more powerful, more precisely focused on the invader, was called for as an extra defence. This was the *immune system*, and it came into being because of the constant threat from microbial and other parasites. It began to be developed early in the evolution of vertebrates, and is precisely focused in the sense that it enables the host to recognize the actual molecules of any invader. The response is directed against these particular foreign molecules, and the memory of the response is stored for future use – imprinted on the immune system. Hence the response to measles virus molecules will defend against measles but not mumps, and because the body remembers the measles response it will resist reinfection with this particular virus at any time in the future. You don't get measles twice.

Special cells take the microbe to pieces and present the pieces to the immune system. As might be expected, the immune system cannot respond to the entire microbe, all in one piece, but does so separately to its various building blocks or molecular components. These are for the most part proteins (large molecules made up of thousands of different amino acids), and they act as *antigens*. An antigen is simply a substance that causes the body to make an immune response to it. The antigens from the microbe are fed into the system ('presented' to it) after being taken up by a special set of *antigen-presenting cells* (APCs). It turns out that the final immune response is made against smaller portions of the protein antigens called *peptides*, which consist of as few as 8–12 amino acid building blocks (see Glossary).

This makes sense because a response to the peptide means a response to the whole protein, which means a response to the microbial invader itself. The antigen-presenting cell therefore digests the microbe's protein down to bite-sized pieces, dissecting out the individual peptides before handing them over (presenting them) to the next cells in the chain of response, the lymphocytes.

Lymphocytes come in two categories, T lymphocytes (T cells from the Thymus) and B lymphocytes (B cells from the Bone marrow). They don't look different but they have vastly different functions. The B cells form antibody, which is a protein that reacts against a particular antigen. As a crude *aide memoire* you can think of anti*body* as produced by the *body*, whereas anti*gens* are the *gen*tlemen coming in from the ouside world. T cells don't secrete antibody but operate in a quite different way, being responsible for what is called cell-mediated immunity (CMI).

The term CMI is a useful one, yet in a sense confusing because all types of immunity are ultimately mediated by cells. But separating off antibody from CMI was the way it happened in the history of immunology (see Box 3), and the distinction between the two remains a real and a useful one. Antibody ('humoral' immunity) and CMI are the two strong arms of the immune system. They work together.

During an infectious disease the body becomes a battlefield, and invading microbes and their antigens may appear at any place, at any time. Immune weapons must be capable of reaching all parts of the body. The B cells live in lymphoid tissues, described below, but the antibody molecules they have formed circulate throughout the body and can act at a distance, independently of the cells that gave birth to them. They are like dust particles in a room, scattered through all spaces, available almost anywhere. CMI, in contrast, depends on local, pinpointed action of T cells, and therefore the T cells themselves must circulate through the body if they are to be ready for action anywhere, as described in Box 4.

Lymphoid organs and lymphoid tissues (Figure 10) are places where lymphocytes meet and interact with each other and with other cells such as APCs and macrophages. It is here that immune responses are set in motion. Lymphoid organs are strategically placed in just those parts of the body where invading microbes are likely to be encountered. Lymph glands in the neck, armpit and groin are ready for invaders from the head, arms and legs, and a massive lymphoid organ, the spleen, monitors and filters the blood that flows through it. A whole ring of lymphoid organs (tonsils and adenoids) surrounds and defends the entrance to the gut and lungs, and additional lymphoid collections are embedded in the gut wall. In child-

Box 3 At loggerheads over antibody and CMI

Emile Adolph von Behring (1814–1917) studied medicine in Berlin, worked in the Robert Koch Institute, and was the one who discovered antibodies. It had recently been demonstrated that a toxic molecule (toxin) was formed by the diphtheria bacterium, and he showed those who had recovered and become resistant to diphtheria had something in their blood serum that neutralized this toxin. He called it an *antikorper* (antibody), a *body* that acted against (*anti*) the toxin. It acted as an antitoxin, and patients could be cured of diphtheria by injection of serum containing this antitoxin. With his colleague Shibasaburo Kitasato he found the same thing to be true for the toxin of tetanus.

In 1901 von Behring was awarded the Nobel Prize, the first one to be given for medicine, and the citation read: 'For his work on serum therapy, especially its application against diphtheria, by which he has opened a new road in the domain of medical science and thereby placed in the hands of the physician a victorious weapon against illness and death.' It was not long before antibodies were also shown to immobilize and kill bacteria. Paul Ehrlich (1854–1915), another Nobel Prize winner, showed that the antibody was bound to the diphtheria toxin and neutralized it because of the shapes of the two molecules. They fitted firmly together, and it was a 'lock and key' interaction, so that the business ends of the toxin molecule were covered up. But many were not convinced that disease resistance was simply a matter of a substance present in blood. What about Metchnikov's phagocytes? (See pages 33–34.) Didn't they kill and digest microbes? And so a fierce battle was waged between those who believed in antibodies and those who favoured cells, although a few scientists, such as Almoth Wright and Stewart Douglas, who in 1903 discovered opsonins, suggested that both mattered. People now began to measure antibodies in the laboratory by their ability to kill, immobilize or agglutinate bacteria. Antibodies were in the limelight, scientists focused on them, and the battle seemed to be won when (between 1939 and 1961) the actual structure of antibodies and their mode of action was worked out.

So CMI languished for want of enthusiasts. In 1950 delayed hypersensitivity reactions in the skin (see Glossary) were described as an expression of CMI, but this discovery could have been made 50 years earlier. The real problem, perhaps, was that CMI seemed more

> **Box 3 At loggerheads over antibody and CMI (continued)**
>
> difficult to study. Several types of cell and many chemical messengers were involved, whereas antibody was a more straightforward chemical matter. It was not until the 1960s that CMI really came into its own and took its rightful place in immunology.

hood, when we first meet and learn how to handle all the common infections, the tonsils and adenoids are often seen to be greatly enlarged when we are asked to say 'Ah'. In the old days they were frequently removed in the belief that they were abnormal, but now we know that they are generally doing a good job.

The antibody and CMI responses that take place in lymphoid organs require co-operation between different types of cell, and a veritable army of cytokines are engaged in chemical conversations between cells. These cytokines have a very local and short-term action. If large amounts are formed they can do damage, and they may spill over into the blood and make you feel ill.

Tailor-made responses to each molecule of an invading microbe are based on the presence of specific recognition sites on lymphocytes. The immune

> **Box 4 The wandering T cell**
>
> When I described the inflammatory response (see Figures 8 and 9) I began by mentioning the normal state of blood vessels in tissues, and noted that occasional white blood cells move through blood vessel walls and enter tissues. The white blood cells that do this are T lymphocytes, and after leaving small blood vessels they crawl over cells, moving through tissues, and make their way to local lymph nodes. Here they join other T cells that have arrived directly from the blood. The T cells leave the node via lymph channels and then re-enter the blood. In this way T cells, which are the prima donnas of the immune system, circulate and recirculate through normal parts of the body, and constantly monitor tissues for the foreign antigens that signify microbial invaders. A given T cell completes the migration circuit about once a day. Nearly all the wandering T cells are of the T helper variety.

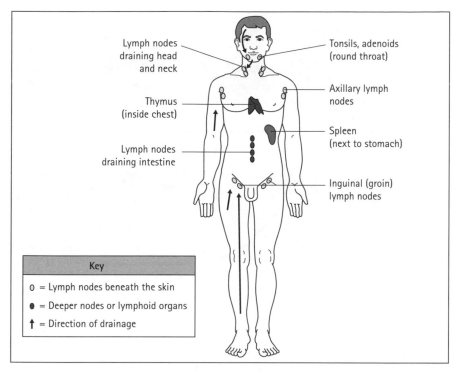

Figure 10 The lymphoid system. The figure shows *visible structures* made up of lymphoid tissue, the headquarters of immune cells. Immune cells are also *scattered* profusely in the skin and in the walls of the respiratory and intestinal tracts.

system gives a precisely focused response to a foreign molecule. The recognition site on the surface of B cells is antibody, and the one on T cells is the T cell's personal receptor (or 'T cell receptor', see below and Figure 11). By means of these sites each T or B cell recognizes one particular molecule (antigen) and can tell it apart from all the others. You may be surprised to hear that when a foreign antigen, whatever it is, enters the body, there will be a few T cells and B cells already present that recognize it. In other words the body has pre-equipped itself with millions of different T and B cells, ready to recognize millions of different antigens. It seems uncanny that Nature has managed to furnish the immune system with all those cells, carrying such a vast range of recognition sites. How is it done? The immunologists have been unravelling these mysteries and have come up with reasonable, though at times complicated, answers.

The T (Thymus) cells are the first to identify and respond to antigens; they

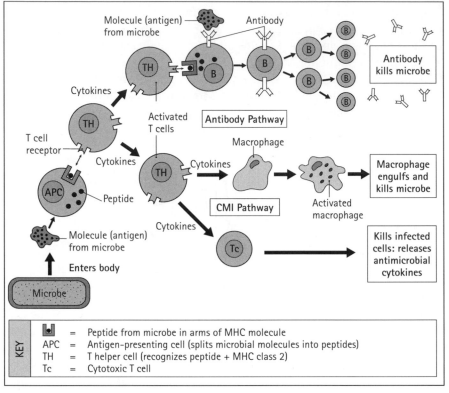

Figure 11 How cells co-operate in an immune response.

are the turnstiles through which all antigens must pass. The exact recognition site displayed on a given T cell is determined by the genes, and there are a hundred or so different genes that look after these sites. During embryonic life a shuffling and reassortment of these genes takes place in each developing lymphocyte, so that a given lymphocyte and its descendants display on their surface a unique receptor which enables them to recognize just one particular antigen. As a result the body contains populations of lymphocytes that can recognize millions of different antigens.

Of course the body does not want to recognize and react with its own molecules (antigens). The power of the immune system is such that a response directed against self could be catastrophic. How does it know what is foreign to the body and what isn't? Decisions about what is foreign and what is 'self' are prearranged in the *thymus gland*. It is here, very early in life, that young T cells are being formed, and those that react with the body's own components are eliminated. These self-reacting cells show their colours at this stage and are then persuaded to commit suicide! (see Apoptosis in Glossary). It is often described as an educational process but really it is a ruthless business, and tens of thousands of young cells perish, the thymus acting as an immunological extermination camp and graveyard.

In this co-ordinated response the self-sacrifice of unwanted immune cells, like the actions of the noble phagocytic warriors that 'die for their country' on the battlefield, remind one of a colony of ants. Survival of the individual cell or ant is irrelevant compared with the wellbeing of the body or the colony as a whole. Yet, in spite of this weeding out process, occasional self-reacting cells slip through, giving rise to what we call *autoimmune diseases* (see Box 5).

How the immune response gets started; calling T cells into action

An immune response gets under way after a T cell has encountered and recognized a foreign antigen. The T cells that do this are the ones that circulate and recirculate through the body (Box 4) and they are called T helper cells. Each T helper cell has its special T cell receptor antennae mounted on the cell surface and projecting from it like antennae. On a given T helper cell the T cell receptor is a recognition site for one particular antigen or antigen fragment (peptide). It recognizes that particular antigen by its shape, and, rather like antibody (Box 3), functions as a lock which only one key will fit perfectly. It may be that the receptor (lock) is never engaged by the right antigen fragment (key) and the T helper cell is never called into action. If the key is inserted into the lock while the T cell is still developing in the thymus gland, surrounded by the body's own molecules, the cell dies rather than matures, as described above, and this is the way in which self-reacting T cells are eliminated. But if it is inserted after the T cell has matured in the thymus, after it has entered the blood and the lymphoid system and is on duty, powerful events are set in motion.

Thus T helper cells set the immune response going, and in doing so act as immunological dictators. When there is something wrong with these cells (for instance in AIDS) the result can be disastrous. The responses to be set in motion are very varied and T helper cells can trigger off (help) either antibody production or cell-mediated responses.

Let us use the zoom lens and examine things in greater detail. The sophistication and precision of the immune response depends on intimate contacts between different types of cells. If you look at Figure 11 you will be able to follow what may seem tortuous but what are in fact logically necessary interactions between cells.

Box 5 Autoimmune diseases

These are diseases caused when immune responses are directed against the body's own components. When such a powerful weapon turns on and attacks the body the consequences can be calamitous. The real miracle is that it happens so rarely.

Autoimmune responses are the basis for diseases such as rheumatoid arthritis, multiple sclerosis, juvenile-type diabetes (the type that starts in childhood and needs insulin), ankylosing spondylitis, probably psoriasis, and a variety of rarer diseases. Luckily most people do not get autoimmune diseases.

Each separate immune response is controlled by genes, and it turns out that the immune response genes are tied up with the genes for a certain set of molecules that label the body's cells. These are the MHC molecules, also known as human leucocyte antigens or HLAs (see Glossary), the ones that are important in organ transplantation. Those who get autoimmune diseases generally have certain types of MHC genes, and this means certain types of immune response genes. For instance those with HLA-A3, B7, or DR2 are more likely to develop multiple sclerosis, which is caused by a T cell immune response to the insulating material round nerve fibres (myelin basic protein).

Many scientists think that autoimmune responses are triggered by microbes. One way in which microbes could do this is when one of their molecules happens to be very similar to a host molecule. The immune system recognizes the microbial material as foreign, and the resulting response to it unfortunately reacts also (cross-reacts) with the host's own tissues. In the course of defeating the microbe the body damages itself. Many common viruses and bacteria have host-like components. Indeed it could be regarded as a sort of microbial strategy (see Part 3). By imitating (mimicking) a host molecule the microbe hopes to reduce the immune response against itself.

We are still a long way from complete understanding of autoimmune diseases, but the idea of an infectious trigger acting in genetically predisposed individuals is a convincing one. These individuals are born with the particular HLAs that go with the self-reactive immune responses.

The fate of a foreign fragment

On entering the body microbial and other foreign antigens are first taken up by macrophages (see pages 34–40), or by large fragile immune cells, called dendritic cells because of their numerous branching processes (Greek, *dendron* = tree). All these are APCs. Because antigens are often large molecules (proteins), the APCs first partially digest the antigen to smaller portions (peptides) which are what the T cells are interested in. Then something special happens. The peptide becomes attached to a special type of MHC molecule (see Glossary) which is present on the surface of the APC, called an MHC class 2 molecule. This molecule, present only on certain immune cells, holds the little peptide firmly in its jaws and it is the whole object, a combination of peptide and MHC, that is offered to T cells.

Why offer peptide plus MHC to the T cell rather than peptide alone? Why complicate matters? The reason is that once the T cell has recognized its antigen it is stimulated and an amazing series of events unfold. The fuse is lit, the immune reaction begins. The T cell needs to ensure that all this takes place in the right part of the body. If it reacted with peptide alone while the latter was floating free in tissues or in the blood the T cell, isolated from other immune cells, could not interact with other cells and could not do its work. It needs to make sure the recognition takes place in the presence of other immune cells, which means in lymphoid tissues. The ideal way to guarantee this is to react with the peptide only when it is combined with the marker, the MHC class 2 molecule, present only on certain immune cells.

The MHC part of the story makes it complicated, and I could have missed it out. But this would have been like describing the workings of a car without mentioning the steering wheel. To return to the unfolding of the immune response, let us assume that among all the T cells that constantly recirculate, moving through tissues and inspecting what is on offer, one will soon turn up that recognizes the particular peptide attached to the MHC class 2 cell marker. It is a momentous event, this first act of recognition, because it tells the body that an invader, which could turn out to be a lethal one, is present.

But the act of recognition has involved only a single T helper cell, and it is therefore on a microscopic scale. Yet the microbe has already begun to multiply and is about to spread through the body, so *the need to magnify the response is urgent*. Therefore, when a T helper cell recognizes its own particular peptide antigen attached to an MHC class 2 molecule on the APC it is stimulated, and it now divides repeatedly to form a clone of tens of thousands of cells with identical reactivity (clonal expansion). Normally only about one in every ten thousand T cells reacts with any given antigen, but during infection with a microbe containing that antigen the proportion increases to about one in a hundred. Unfortunately cell division is a complicated process and takes at least eight hours. Hence it is not for nearly a week that enough of the right cells have been produced to give real power to the response. *It is because of this inescapable delay in the immune response that the early defences are so crucial.*

Another problem with the T cell's act of recognition is that it takes place in one corner of the body, say under the skin of a finger or in the lymph node up in the armpit. There is therefore an urgent need to broadcast the response through the body, because the microbe itself may soon spread through the body. Accordingly, many of the stimulated and newly formed clones of T cells enter lymphatics, reach the blood, and are disseminated throughout the body.

Each stimulated T helper cell can start off either an antibody or a cell-mediated immune response, as outlined in Figure 11. Let us now see what happens after a T helper cell has been stimulated and sets off an antibody response.

B lymphocytes are the producers of antibody, and each cell can turn into an antibody factory, making one predetermined type of antibody. Every B cell is coated with a thin layer of the antibody it is destined to make, a sample of what it can produce.

The initial recognition has been made by a T helper cell, and it must now find a B cell that is scheduled to make an antibody reacting with the same peptide, and help it to do so. How does it recognize the right B cell? This B cell would have been displaying on its surface a sample of the antibody it can produce, and has probably already used it to trap the antigen, plugging the antigen into itself by a lock and key mechanism. But if this act of recognition has happened, why can't the B cell just get on with the job without delay and form its antibody? Why have yet another time-consuming complication? The reason is that if this were all that were needed to start off antibody production there would be unnecessary, unsuitable stimulation of a wider range of B cells, which are surrounded by the body's own molecules. Self-reacting antibodies would be formed. Remember that these cells, unlike the T cells, have not been educated in the thymus, and they do not know about not responding to self antigens. The B cell that has trapped its antigen therefore needs to get an 'OK' from the immunological dictator, the T cell.

So that the B cell can speak the T cell's peptide language it digests the trapped antigen to peptide and displays it on its surface in the arms of an

MHC class 2 molecule, just like a regular APC. The B cell now waits. It is ready to respond, but only if the appropriate T cell touches it, recognizes it and tells it to do so. Once this second recognition event has taken place the B cell does its stuff. It enlarges, divides repeatedly to form large numbers of offspring all forming exactly the same antibody (another example of *clonal expansion*), and then begins to convert itself into an antibody factory, producing up to 10,000 antibody molecules a minute. Because cell division takes time (a minimum of eight hours) it is not until several days later that worthwhile amounts of antibody have been formed.

As can be imagined, much movement of cells is needed if all these specific assignations are to be made. During an immune response the body's lymphoid organs (spleen, lymph nodes) are a seething mass of cells, which are searching for appropriate collaborators. The search is made easier because particular responses, such as antibody production, take place in designated areas of lymphoid organs. The cells move over one another, tirelessly checking for surface labels, some of them migrating in the lymph and blood to distant parts of the body. When the right contacts have been made, the immunological dialogue begins with the exchange of various chemical messages as summarized in Figure 14, and the B cells can now fulfil their destiny. They start making their antibodies.

A different sequence of events is set in motion when a T helper cell is stimulated and sets off a cell-mediated immune response. In this case (Figure 11) the stimulated T helper cell releases a different set of chemical messages from those used for antibodies, and the result is a CMI response. This entails activation of macrophages, and formation of a separate type of T cell, the *cytotoxic T cell*, whose antimicrobial action is described on page 65. We are not sure what it is that makes a T helper cell go down the CMI rather than the antibody pathway, but local pulses of cytokines (especially one called interleukin-12) have a lot to do with it. Although these two strong arms of immunity act together, either one or the other may be more helpful to the host in a given infection. For instance, a good cell-mediated response means you recover from tuberculosis, whereas in this particular infection a mainly antibody response is bad news.

Antibodies and how they do their job

Antibodies were discovered in the 1890s, and much of their structure and mode of action was worked out in the 1920s–1950s. We know a lot about them. It took much longer for the intricacies of cell-mediated immunity to be unravelled, and we were still adding to the picture in the 1980s and 1990s.

The structure of antibody

The basic antibody (referred to as immunoglobulin or Ig) molecule is in the shape of a Y. Antibodies can be life-saving and the Y shape, suggesting that Yes, I can protect you, do this and do that for you, is perhaps appropriate! On the upper ends of the Y are the parts that react with the antigen. They have a complementary shape to the antigen, and fit it rather like a key fits a lock. As an example of this specificity, human serum albumin injected into a rabbit will induce the formation of antibodies that react with human serum albumin but not with the serum albumin of cows, chickens or mice.

Antibodies may be needed in any part of the body (blood, intestine, vagina) and to accommodate this requirement there are several types or classes of antibody, each designed to function under different circumstances. All are made up of the same basic Y shape, and it is the part of the molecule situated on the stem of the Y that gives the antibody its class and its biological functions.

- *Class G (IgG) antibodies are the main antibodies in the blood.* G for General workhorse antibodies. They consist of the basic Y-shaped structure. They leak out into tissues quite easily, and small amounts are normally found, for instance in the fluid (cerebrospinal fluid) surrounding the brain.

- *Class A (IgA) antibody is exported onto mucosal surfaces.* A for Acting at surfaces. It is made up of two of the basic Y-shaped molecules, and called secretory antibody because it is secreted onto the mucosal surfaces of the alimentary, respiratory, urinary and genital tracts. Here it is in a fine position to act directly on invading microbes. It is also secreted into milk (see Glossary), especially into colostrum, the first formed milk, and helps protect the infant against many intestinal infections. We can see the critical importance of the mucosal scene by noting that in the wall of the intestine, for instance, there are altogether about ten thousand million B cells that form IgA antibody, some of them actually engaged in immune responses, many others poised and ready for action. The gut is the body's biggest battlefield.

- *Class M (IgM) is a very large type of antibody, present in blood.* M for Massive. Each molecule is made up of five of the basic Y-shaped molecules. This means that it has five times as many sites that can combine with antigen, making IgM, molecule for molecule, much more powerful than IgG or IgA. Because of its large size it cannot easily pass through blood vessel walls, so it stays in the blood. Why has Nature produced this extra type of antibody? Surely not for the confusion of students or the delight of immunologists! The answers are given in Box 6.

Box 6 Why do we have IgM antibodies?

(Items 2–4 are explanations rather than reasons)

1. It is a *powerful* type of antibody. Each molecule of IgM antibody consists of five of the basic Y-shaped molecules and therefore has five times the power of a molecule of IgG.

2. It is *first* to appear in an immune response, a day or two before IgG. This time difference can be crucial because in every infection there is a *race* between multiplication of the invading microbe and the appearance on the scene of defensive antibodies. As the response unfolds the IgM are replaced by IgG antibodies. The switch to IgG has practical applications. If a pregnant woman is suspected of having been infected with rubella (German measles) virus her blood can be tested for IgM antibody to rubella. If it is present you know that the infection was recent or is still in progress, but if she has only IgG antibody she was probably infected at some time in the past.

3. It is *first* to appear in the development of the individual, in the fetus. This too has practical consequences. When a pregnant woman is infected with rubella or cytomegalovirus (two viruses that cause birth defects) she forms IgG antibodies which pass across the placenta to the fetus and can be detected in the blood of the newborn infant. If the newborn infant has IgG antibodies to rubella or cytomegalovirus it merely signifies that the mother has at some time been infected. If, however, the fetus itself has been infected it will have formed its own IgM antibodies. Maternal IgM are too large to pass across placental blood vessels to the fetus, so that if they are present in the infant's blood it means that the infant has made these antibodies and was therefore infected *in utero*. In this way the cause of birth defects can be ascertained.

4. It is *first* to appear in the evolution of vertebrates. It is the type of antibody seen in primitive fishes, whereas IgG is a more recent invention, appearing with the mammals.

- *Class E (IgE) antibody is responsible for allergic reactions.* E for Explosive. As far as amounts are concerned it is a very minor type of antibody, and it is formed by B cells lying just below the respiratory and intestinal surfaces. It attaches itself to special cells in these sites called mast cells, and should it then meet and react with antigen from a parasitic worm, for instance, the mast cell is stimulated to release a pulse of histamine. The histamine causes a local reaction that helps expel the worm from the intestine. Unfortunately the same IgE response that is useful for dealing with worms also gives rise to hayfever, asthma, and (in the skin) eczema. In a hayfever sufferer the reaction takes place after inhaling things like pollens or substances from house mites, which act as the antigen (allergen). The local mast cells now release histamine and other substances, and this causes a running nose and itchy eyes, or a stomach-ache if the offending allergen has been eaten. Very occasionally IgE is responsible for a more severe reaction, for instance in people exquisitely sensitive to bee or wasp venom or to peanuts. This is called anaphylaxis, and is treated by injecting adrenalin.

More about antibodies

Our blood (or serum) contains a vast assortment of different antibodies, of different classes and directed against tens of thousands of different antigens. Twenty per cent of all the protein in the blood is antibody, and it is a mixed bag. When a microbial invader multiplies and forms its foreign antigens, large numbers of different B cells are stimulated. Each form an antibody directed against a single one of the many microbial components (antigens). A stimulated B cell also divides repeatedly to form descendants, and therefore the body soon contains different populations of B cells, each forming its own sort of antibody, directed against one of the antigens, and belonging to a certain class.

By the time we reach adult life all of us have been exposed to a wide variety of infectious agents, have produced antibody to them, and have remembered those responses. If the same microbe enters the body again fresh supplies of the relevant antibody can rapidly be formed. Antibody is the main immunological gift that a mother can give to her child, other than a collection of good immune response genes. Her IgG antibodies leak through the placenta to the fetus and protect the newborn infant for several months against a great variety of common infections. An additional valuable donation comes in the form of her IgA antibodies present in milk (colostrum).

The magic of monoclonal antibody

Immunology took a great step forwards in 1975 when two immunologists, George Kohler and Cesar Milstein, discovered how to make monoclonal antibodies. They were awarded the Nobel Prize for this feat.

As we have seen, a given B cell and its descendants form antibody, which is directed against one particular antigen and is of one particular class. Therefore when a single antibody-producing cell is separated from all the others, isolated in a test tube, and encouraged to divide, it produces a 'clone' of millions of descendants. The antibody they form is all of exactly the same class and reactivity, and is called monoclonal antibody. Monoclonal antibodies, the immunological equivalent of pure chemicals, have been of extraordinary value in immunology and medicine.

Testing for antibodies

Antibodies are easily tested for in the laboratory, and when they are present in blood serum it means that the microbe in question has at some time been encountered. Other questions may need to be answered. Are the antibodies present because the patient has at some time been vaccinated against that microbe, or have they been formed in response to an actual infection? Are they of the IgM class, signifying a recent or current infection? The actual amount of antibody present can be checked (titrated) in the laboratory, and this enables the physician to compare serum taken at the onset of the illness with that taken a week or two later. An increase means that the patient has just been infected. Using this method, or by testing for IgM antibodies, the diagnosis can be made.

How antibodies help the host fight the invader

Antibodies are formed against most of the different components (antigens) of a microbe. The larger microbes, naturally, have a larger number of components; more than a thousand for a bacterium compared with less than ten for a small virus. But not all the antibodies are useful to the host. Some will react with unimportant parts of the microbe and have no influence on the infection; others will be of poor quality, making a bad fit with the antigen.

Exactly how do antibodies benefit the host, protecting against disease and eventually helping eliminate the invader? The most useful ones are those that react either with the outer surface of the microbe or with key microbial enzymes and toxins. These particular antibodies are useful because the outer surface of the microbe is directly exposed to attack, because enzymes are needed by the microbe when it multiplies, and because the microbial toxins cause damage.

Antibodies in action – the six special things (see Figure 12)
It may seem confusing, but antibodies act in six different ways. Yet the fact that they do so is fortunate because different microbes need different treatment. An antibody action suitable for one may be unsuitable for another. Also, as mentioned earlier, microbes have come up with answers to many of these actions, and it pays the immune system to keep alternative methods of defence up its sleeve. There is a degree of redundancy in the system. In any case, attacking an invader by several methods at the same time makes good military sense.

1. Antibodies prevent the microbe attaching to the host cell
Many microbes (see Part 3) have surface molecules that stick them onto host cells, and this attachment is a necessary step in invasion. If the attachment molecules of influenza virus or the gonococcus, for instance, are coated with antibody, attachment and invasion is prevented. The invader is halted in its tracks.

2. Antibodies act as opsonins
The pneumococcus is one of the commonest causes of pneumonia. This bacterium has a slimy (polysaccharide) coat, nicely designed to make phagocytosis difficult. As seen in the test tube a polymorph phagocyte trying to engulf one of these bacteria finds that it slips out if its ineffective grip like a wet fish. When as few as ten pneumococci are introduced into the peritoneal cavity of a mouse the animal dies, unable to control their growth. Yet when the pneumococci are coated by antibody (directed against the polysaccharide coat) the result is dramatically different. In the test tube the polymorphs ingest the bacteria with consummate ease, and now at least 10,000 bacteria must be introduced into the peritoneal cavity to have a lethal effect. The antibody gives that great gift – enhanced phagocytosis of bacteria, and increased resistance to infection.

How do antibodies have such a striking effect on phagocytosis? After antibody molecules have attached to the microbe's surface, grasping it by the arms of the Y, the stems are left projecting outwards. Phagocytes are equipped with surface molecules that combine specifically with the stem of the antibody. As the approaching phagocyte encounters the forest of antibody stems sticking out from the microbe it attaches to them, and phagocytosis is triggered off. The microbe is engulfed, killed and digested, as in Figure 8, and this occurs much faster and more completely than would have been possible without antibody. It is as if the microbe has been covered with a red paint, easily recognized by the phagocyte. Instead of sticking to a

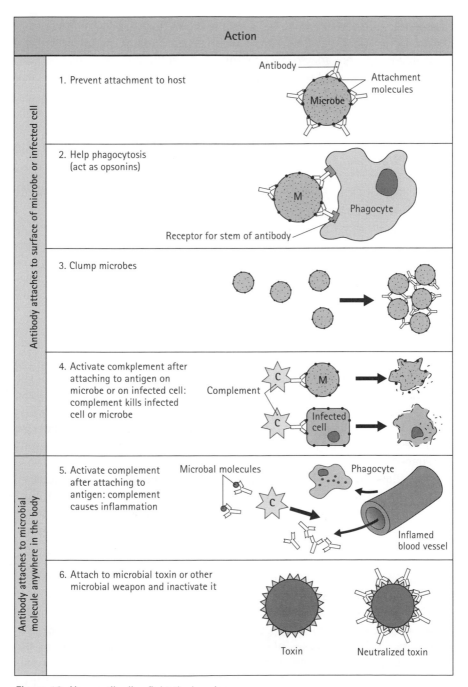

Figure 12 How antibodies fight the invader.

susceptible host cell the microbe is now stuck to the phagocyte and is soon locked in its lethal embrace. Acting in this way, making the microbe more palatable for the phagocyte, more easily eaten, antibody functions as a kind of sauce or seasoning. Such antibodies are therefore called 'opsonins' (Greek = sauce or seasoning).

George Bernard Shaw was a close friend of Sir Almroth Wright who, together with his colleague at St Mary's Hospital, London, Dr Stewart Douglas, discovered opsonins in 1903. In the Preface of his play, *The Doctor's Dilemma*, Shaw says: 'The white corpuscles or phagocytes, which attack and devour disease germs for us, do their work only when we butter the disease germ appetizingly for them with a natural sauce which Sir Almroth named opsonin...'.

I should add that the opsonic action is further increased because of complement. When antibody reacts with microbial antigen, complement joins in the reaction and is activated (see 4, below). Phagocytes have receptors that stick onto the activated portions of complement (as well as receptors for the stem of the antibody, as described above), and the opsonization process is enhanced.

3. Antibodies clump microbes
In one of the early tests for antibodies, used on patients with suspected typhoid, the serum to be tested was mixed with typhoid bacteria and if the bacteria formed visible clumps then antibody was present. Antibodies clump the bacteria together (agglutinate them) by attaching to them and forming bridges between them. This is good for the host because when 10 separate microbes are clumped into one single mass the number of infectious units is reduced ten-fold.

Antibodies can also 'paralyse' the microbe, stopping it moving about if, like cholera or leptospira bacteria, it is the sort that can do this. But most bacteria, and certainly all viruses, are not mobile and don't move about under their own steam, so antibodies that immobilize have a limited sphere of action.

4. Antibodies activate the complement system, which can then punch holes in the microbe
Wherever it occurs, attachment of antibody to its antigen starts off a chain of events called 'complement activation' as outlined in Box 7. When the activation takes place on the microbe's surface, some of the substances formed from complement make holes in this surface. Materials leak out through the holes and the microbe dies. If the microbial antigen

---

Box 7 Complement and how it helps antibody

The word complement refers to a collection of about 30 different molecules that are present in the blood in an inactive form. Activation of the first of its molecules (called C1) sets off a train of events of immense importance for defence against microbes.

The initial recognition by antibody of a foreign antigen is an exceedingly small-scale local event. But it sets off an alarm and (like the recognition of foreign antigen by a T cell) it may signal the beginning of a serious infection. As soon as possible it must be amplified into something larger and more powerful. This is where complement comes in. The reaction of antibody with antigen lights the fuse for the complement gunpowder. The first molecule to be activated (C1) activates many more molecules of the next one in the series, and this in turn forms even larger numbers of the next molecule, and so on. It is a snowball effect, a chain reaction, and the freshly activated molecules do useful things, such as helping phagocytosis (see Item 2, page 60), causing inflammation (see Item 5), and killing the microbe (see Item 4, page 62). Like the clotting system and the immune system as a whole, it may harm the host if it is triggered off inappropriately. Therefore it contains mechanisms for controlling itself and switching itself off.

The complement system can also be set off without antibody having to react with antigen. As mentioned in Chapter 2, certain molecules on the surface of bacteria (polysaccharides and endotoxin) as well as on viruses and other microbes, can set it off on their own. This is an ancient method of defence, part of what we called the *early defences*, and was used by primitive animals long before antibodies were invented. The potent complement molecules were later recruited to help with immune defences.

---

is on the surface of a host cell the same thing happens and the cell is killed.

5. Antibodies activate the complement system, which then causes inflammation

Setting off the complement system (with or without antibody) also leads to the release of molecules that cause inflammation. Inflammation, by attracting phagocytes and antibodies to the affected area (see pages 30–33), is generally useful to the host.

6. Antibodies neutralize microbial toxins

When antibody combines with the sort of microbial antigen that acts as a toxin, or with a microbial molecule that interferes with host defences, it neutralizes its action. This is clearly valuable for the host.

On Christmas Eve in Berlin in 1891 a small child lay dying with diphtheria. The bacteria (*Corynebacterium diphtheriae*) had become established in the throat and larynx and were liberating their special toxin. The thick layer of dead tissue that had formed locally was interfering with breathing, and the toxin was also having harmful effects on the heart and nervous system. Dr Heinrich Giessler, the physician, had managed to obtain some antibody, in the form of blood serum taken from laboratory rabbits injected with the toxin, and this was infused into the child's vein. By the next morning the breathing was less laboured, and the child recovered. The bacterial toxin had been neutralized. Before the days of antibiotics, antitoxins (antibodies in the serum of horses) were widely used to treat diseases like diphtheria, caused by toxin-forming bacteria.

The cell-mediated response and how it does its job

T helper cells activate macrophages

One of the most powerful chemical messengers to come from the stimulated T helper cell is *interferon gamma*. This key chemical acts on macrophages, which are normally in a relaxed ('resting') state. Interferon gamma asks them to switch on their antimicrobial powers and have all their weapons formed and ready. The macrophages respond by developing greatly enhanced power to phagocytose, kill, and digest the invaders. You can see the change in the test tube. The activated macrophages not only take up foreign particles with greater enthusiasm but they also, in a valiant attempt to phagocytose the test tube itself, spread out and attach so firmly to the glass surface that you can only dislodge them by scraping them off. A very simple substance, nitric oxide (not to be confused with nitrous oxide or 'laughing gas', used in anaesthesia) is one of the substances they form which accounts for their enhanced killing power (see Figure 8).

Macrophages are vital cells in defence, not only against the general run of microbes, but also against microbes that live in cells, such as tuberculosis bacteria and viruses; indeed macrophages themselves are frequently invaded. When the T helper cell arms them in this way it gives the host a vital boost in the battle with the invader. This response, therefore, increases the fighting strength of a key soldier on the battlefield. It can be compared with the antibodies that increase the fighting strength of that other soldier, the polymorph (see page 40).

In the cell-mediated response there is another type of T cell, the cytotoxic T cell, that can kill other cells

Cytotoxic T cells are programmed to recognize foreign peptide antigens (generally viral) that have been formed in infected cells and have been displayed on the cell surface in the arms of MHC class 1 molecules. The latter are distinct from the MHC class 2 molecules referred to earlier in this chapter, and the reason for their participation at this stage is explained in Box 8. The cytotoxic T cell, once it has encountered and recognized the foreign antigen on the infected cell, is now stimulated and proceeds to kill it. It does this either by switching on the target cell's own suicide programme (see below) or by inserting into the target cell wall a special molecule (perforin) that makes holes in it. The contents of the target cell then leak out and it dies, the debris being cleared up by phagocytes. Although the victim is a living host cell, the foreign peptide antigen on its surface has labelled it as infected by a virus, and this means it is soon going to release hundreds of virus offspring. It must be destroyed before the virus has finished multiplying, and the body shows no hesitation in killing off its own cells under these circumstances. The few must be sacrificed for the sake of the whole. Cytotoxic T cells are important in defence whether or not they actually kill infected cells because they also release cytokines that do other useful things such as interfere with the multiplication of viruses.

Microbes have forced the host to make another type of killer cell – the natural killer (NK) cell

The cytotoxic T cell is a serious threat to microbes that live in cells, such a threat that many of them have responded by interfering with the display of the MHC class 1 molecules that the cytotoxic T cell must recognize on the target cell surface (see also Part 3). Such a cell can now no longer be identified and killed because the microbial peptide on its own is not enough. This sounds like a winning strategy for the microbe. But the host in turn has replied by forming a special sort of T cell, the NK cell, which recognizes and kills any cells that *don't* have the usual MHC class 1 label! The NK cell does not worry about foreign antigens, but identifies and kills any cell without MHC class 1, using the same methods as the cytotoxic T cell. Any cell without MHC class 1 is assumed to be infected and is killed. Another microbial strategy is thereby foiled.

Box 8   Care is needed when switching on a cytotoxic T cell's lethal weapons

What the cytotoxic T cell actually recognizes is the antigen (peptide) attached to an MHC class 1 molecule. The small peptide is sitting snugly in a groove on the surface of the large MHC class 1 molecule, and these molecules are present on all cells in the body. Remember that it is the MHC class 2 molecules that are present only on APC and B cells. One of the great leaps forward in immunology was when in 1972 Peter Doherty and Rolf Zinkernagel, working in Canberra, Australia, found that these MHC class 1 molecules, known to be important in the transplantation of organs between individuals (see Box 5), were also fundamental for cytotoxic T cell responses. Cytotoxic T cells would only kill cells that had been infected with a virus if they recognized on them not only the peptide antigen of the virus, but also their own MHC class 1 molecules. Each individual has different MHC class 1 molecules. Cytotoxic T cells do not kill the target cell in spite of its display of the relevant antigen if it is from an unrelated individual; the MHC class 1 molecule is now different and it is not recognized. For this discovery the two scientists were awarded the Nobel Prize.

But why is this so complicated? Why has Nature evolved this seemingly difficult system of recognition? A moment's reflection will show that it makes sense. If the cytotoxic T cell recognized the peptide by itself, perhaps floating free or temporarily attached to an innocent uninfected cell, it would lead to undesirable and inappropriate results. The cytotoxic weapons and the cytokines would then be discharged uselessly into the extracellular fluids of the body, or perhaps onto a harmless bystander cell. MHC class 1 molecules, however, are present on the surface of all cells in the body, and because it is forced to recognize these molecules as well as the peptide antigen the cytotoxic T cell only fires off its weapons when it is actually in contact with another cell. The target cell is usually infected with a virus, and indeed can be regarded as having made this display with an altruistic, self-sacrificing motive.

Cell suicide

The eternal sequence of host defence, microbial response and host counter-response, as set out in Section 3, is further illustrated by cell suicide. When a cell is infected by a virus it becomes a mere assembly line for the virus unless it is identified early enough and killed. One defence strategy would be for the cell to autodestruct once it had been infected. Infected cells generally die but it is sometimes hard to lay the blame directly on the virus, and there are some viruses, moreover, that do little or no damage to the cell. As often as not the cell dies by switching on its own in-built suicide programme, called *apoptosis* (see Glossary). Cells need to have such a programme because apoptosis is a feature of normal embryology and cell renewal. Our tail, quite prominent in the early fetus, is later remoulded and reduced, just like the tail of a tadpole as it turns into a frog. A certain amount of destruction accompanies construction! The same programme is called into action once a cell is infected with a virus that would not by itself be lethal. It can be regarded as a defence device in which the cell, for the benefit of the whole, autodestructs rather than allows itself to continue as a virus factory. Faced with this tactic many viruses, such as hepatitis B, adenoviruses and Epstein–Barr (EB) virus, have responded by interfering with the apoptosis programme.

Memory

After the first encounter with a microbial antigen it takes a week or more for antibodies and T cell immunity to come into action and control the infection. This is mostly because cell division is a time-consuming business. Afterwards, when the B and T cells have done their job, their numbers decrease, but the body is left with more of those particular B and T cells than originally. They are also more easily switched on. If the microbial antigen now reappears on the scene the response (the *secondary response*) is therefore greater and now takes only a few days. As a result the microbe either fails to infect or is eliminated at an early stage. This is referred to as 'immunological memory'. It lasts at least ten years, and nearly half of our wandering, recirculating T cells carry memory of previous encounters. As with other types of memory it is of immense value. In adult life we are no longer susceptible to measles, mumps, and a host of other infectious ailments, thanks to our memory T cells.

Summary of the immune response

This completes the account of immune defences. In summary, the T helper cells are the eyes and ears of the immune defences and their job is to recognize foreign intruders. Once they have done so they switch on a formidable piece of machinery. A hail of bullets and arrows is released (antibody) and front-line soldiers (phagocytes) and other specialist combat units (cytotoxic T cells) are mobilized and armed. The attack on the invader begins.

Summary 1 – Setting up an immune response (see also Figure 11)

Microbe enters body and one of its antigens is
   engulfed by an APC (antigen-presenting cell)
   and *digested* to a smaller molecule (peptide)
   and *displayed* or 'presented' (with MHC class 2*) on the APC's surface.

Wandering T helper cell capable of recognizing this particular peptide/MHC class 2
   encounters the APC, and
   recognizes it by means of the T cell receptor (special recognition site on T helper cell)

T helper cell is now stimulated, and divides repeatedly (to amplify the response), and either:

1. R*eleases cytokines* that turn resting macrophages into aggressive microbe-killers,

and

causes formation of the type of T cells *(cytotoxic T cells)* that kill infected host cells and form antimicrobial substances

This is cell-mediated immunity (CMI)

or   2. Finds a B cell displaying the same peptide/MHC class 2

recognizes it by means of the T cell receptor and

switches on the B cell which divides repeatedly and all the offspring form antibody

This is the antibody arm of the response

* The peptide is carried as a cargo in the arms of an MHC class 2 molecule (see text).

The two summary tables outline:
1. The events during the setting up of an immune response, and
2. The methods by which the immune response protects us.

Summary 2 – How immune defences protect the host

Antibody
1. Prevents the microbe *attaching* to cells and invading them.
2. Marks the microbe as ready for destruction by phagocytes; the opsonic kiss of death.
3. Clumps the microbes.
4. Marks the microbe (or the infected cell) as ready for killing by complement.
5. Reacts with microbial antigen and sets off the complement system, causing inflammation.
6. Sticks to microbial toxins and neutralizes their harmful effect.

Cell-mediated immunity (CMI)

There are only two items on this list, but these are the tall twin towers of cell-mediated immune defence, which is vital for dealing with microbes that invade cells.

1. Helper T cells turn resting macrophages into efficient killing machines.

2. Cytotoxic T cells recognize cells infected by viruses or other intracellular microbes, and either kill them or release substances that inhibit multiplication of the microbe.

Chapter 4

CHINKS IN THE ARMOUR; THINGS THAT GO WRONG WITH OUR DEFENCES

Amusing organ causes trouble

It was 1965, and Richard, aged 21, had been riding motor cycles for nearly three years. In fine weather there was no better way to travel, the power surging between the knees, the air rushing past, the way you could filter through traffic holdups. He kept the bike in good condition, loved its gleaming contours, and it was cheap to run. Once, on a rainy day, he had skidded and come off, bruising his arm, but that was all.

Statistics tell us that young motor cyclists have a greater risk of accidents than young car drivers. Two wheels are not so safe as four. In November 1965 the statistics caught up with Richard. Coming round a bend in a country road he met a slow-moving tractor and hit it head on. In hospital his fractured femur and ribs were attended to, but he was still in a critical state, and it was decided he was bleeding into the abdomen. When he opened it the surgeon saw that the blood was coming from a badly torn and lacerated spleen. There was nothing for it but to remove the spleen, and Richard then made an uneventful recovery. The motor cycle had been badly damaged, and his girlfriend made him buy a car instead.

The next winter, following what seemed like a bad cold and bronchitis, he suddenly became very ill and was taken to hospital. It was pneumonia, and pneumococcal bacteria were recovered from his lungs and blood. He was treated with antibiotics and recovered.

Pneumococcal pneumonia is uncommon in young adults, and causes problems mostly in the very young and the very old, but Richard was especially susceptible. The spleen is the main source of antibodies, and without it he could not produce enough of them to control the invading bacteria. It is opsonic antibodies (see pages 60–62) that are vital for resisting bacteria like pneumococci and, deprived of opsonic help, his phagocytes could not take up and kill these particular invaders.

In the late 1970s a vaccine for pneumococci came out, and after several injections Richard formed enough antibodies to protect him against further infection. Luckily he has not had trouble with the other bacterial infections (*Haemophilus influenzae* and meningococci) where opsonic antibodies are needed.

Each individual reacts differently to an infection. Inoculate ten people with an identical dose of the same microbe and you will see ten different diseases. This is because the outcome of an infection depends not only on the microbe (the 'seed') but also on the 'soil' (the host). Put crudely, it takes two, the seed and the soil, to make an infection or a disease. In this chapter we will see how the host (the 'soil') influences the outcome of an infection.

Our defences are by no means unchangeable. Their quality and strength differ in different individuals, and any defects have an impact on susceptibility to infectious disease. Defects range from a cut on the skin temporarily allowing the entry of microbes, to an inherited defect in phagocytes or the immune system that may prove to be fatal. In a given person the defences will fluctuate according to age, hormones, nutrition and stress, and people also show genetic (constitutional) differences in defences.

In addition, we will try to answer the question as to which defences matter most. One of the best ways of assessing the importance of each type of defence is to see what happens when it goes wrong. In the words of the early physiologists, 'If an organ puzzles you, take it out and see what happens.'

FAULTY SURFACE DEFENCES

Defects in the surface barriers and in the cleansing mechanisms (see Figure 6) are classic causes of trouble.

Skin
Wounds in the skin get contaminated with bacteria that normally live on the skin (Figure 17), as well as by any that were on the object that caused the wound or that originated from the soil. Even clean wounds made by the surgeon are inevitably contaminated, but they do not usually cause trouble unless harmful bacteria are present or the wound is in the vicinity of that bacteriological factory, the bowel. Harmful strains of streptococcus

bacteria, for instance, very occasionally cause an alarming condition called *necrotizing fasciitis*. The bacteria enter at the site of a local injury or after a minor operation, and spread rapidly under the skin and along the spaces between the muscle bundles (Latin, *fascia* = bundle). A day or so later the patient becomes ill and areas of gangrene (the word means the eating away or death of tissues) are appearing in the affected muscles and overlying skin. As the invading bacteria multiply and spread life is threatened, and there is nothing for it but to cut away all the dead tissues ruthlessly, and give antibiotics. The condition is rare, but it has been given undue prominence by being referred to in the media as caused by a *flesh-eating bug*.

After bad *burns*, skin bacteria that are normally harmless are suddenly presented with golden opportunities, and they colonize and multiply in the damaged areas. The damaged areas provide a highly nutritious surface, and what's more the burn itself causes upsets in the immune system and in the function of phagocytes.

Skin defences are breached whenever an injection is given or when fluids such as blood are infused into veins, although the actual wound is small and rarely causes trouble. On the other hand these needles or injected fluids may be contaminated with microbes which are then inadvertently introduced into the body. In this way people get infected with hepatitis viruses or with HIV.

Skin defences are also weakened when there are general body defects, for instance in the blood circulation (diabetes), or in the immune system and phagocytes.

Skin is best defended if it is *dry*. When feet are encased in socks and shoes the skin stays moist and soft, and various fungi then have the opportunity to invade the dead outer layers. About one in ten of shod human beings have athelete's foot, due to fungi colonizing the skin areas between the toes. But shoes give protection against thorns and other injuries, and in tropical Africa, where unpleasant types of fungi can then penetrate the skin, the unshod are at a disadvantage.

Respiratory tract

The mucosal surfaces of the nose, throat and lungs are often damaged by viruses. The viruses that do this are specialist invaders and establish themselves in spite of normally operating defences (see Part 4). The damaged mucosa now becomes colonized by resident bacteria such as staphylococci and streptococci (see page 137). During a common cold the fluid running from the nose is at first fairly clear, as the infecting virus multiplies. But it soon turns whiter and thicker, because it then contains the colonizing bacteria plus the army of polymorphs that has been called to the scene. When it happens lower down, in the chest, a mild viral illness can turn into bacterial bronchitis or pneumonia, and the patient needs to be given antibiotics.

In normal people the steady flow of mucus over the respiratory surfaces (the mucociliary escalator) is a valuable part of defence. Problems with mucus are seen in the disease *cystic fibrosis*. It is an inherited disease, and as many as one person in 20 carries the gene for it, although only about one in 2500 get the disease. Mucus-producing cells are abnormal and the lungs contain thick, sticky mucus that seriously interferes with the action of cilia. The mucus cannot be moved along and resident bacteria can start an infection. The outlook is ominous if that harmful bacterium *Pseudomonas aeruginosa* (see Glossary) arrives on the scene.

Urinary and genital tracts

The urinary passages are normally kept clean by the flow of urine, but they become susceptible to infection when this flushing action is interfered with. In the elderly male, for instance, an enlarged prostate gland prevents complete emptying of the bladder, and a sump of urine is left behind in which bacteria eventually become established and cause a urinary infection (cystitis). Not unexpectedly, pushing a catheter up the urethra introduces bacteria into the bladder. The catheter also interferes with the flushing action of urine, and if it is left in place for more than a day or so infection is almost guaranteed. If bacteria from the bowel get a foothold near the opening of the female urethra, the mechanical action of the penis can push the infection into the urethra and bladder. Cystitis is commoner in sexually active women.

FAULTY PHAGOCYTES

The vital defence role of the phagocyte is illustrated by the fact that infections soon begin to trouble a person when the number of polymorphs in the blood falls from the normal $2-5 \times 10^9$ per litre to less than 10^9 per litre.

Inherited defects in the phagocyte are rare but they have dramatic effects. Children with *chronic granulomatous disease* have polymorphs that can move about and phagocytose as normal, but cannot then kill the bacteria they have engulfed. One of the key enzymes for forming the antibacterial oxygen radicals in the cell (Figure 11) is missing. In spite of the fact that other defences, including immune responses, are intact the patient suffers repeated infections with normally harmless bacteria like *Escherichia coli* and staphylococci, and usually dies during childhood.

FAULTY IMMUNE RESPONSE

A person with weak immune responses or who makes the wrong type of response is generally in trouble with infections. Death is the eventual penalty for serious deficiences. This is because the *early defences* are not by themselves enough to deal with many microbial invaders. We recover so easily, so unwittingly, from most infections that we take our immune powers for granted. Their life-saving function is made apparent when we see what happens to people with immune handicaps. Most people with severe immune defects are in hospitals, protected by modern medicine and technology. Fifty years ago they would have died, overwhelmed by infection, victims of microbes that are normally kept at bay. From these unfortunate patients we also get an idea of the role of each of the two arms of the immune response.

Antibodies
Children are sometimes born with a condition called *agammaglobulinaemia*. This means that they are unable to form antibodies, but their cell-mediated immunity (CMI) responses are normal. These children suffer repeated infection with the bacteria (pneumococci, *H. influenzae*) that have to be opsonized (see pages 61–62) before they can be phagocytosed and killed. They also have difficulty controlling one or two virus infections. Poliomyelitis virus, if it is to cause paralysis, must leave the intestine and travel in the blood to reach the nervous system. Normally, as soon as it gets into the blood it is inactivated by antibody. When children with severe agammaglobulinaemia are given live poliomyelitis virus vaccine (Sabin type), which multiplies in the intestine, they fail to form antibodies. This means that if the virus enters the blood there is now nothing to stop it travelling to the brain. Such children are 10,000 times more likely than normal children to develop paralysis.

The spleen is a fine filter of blood but it is also an important source of antibody. People who have lost their spleen, for instance in an automobile accident (see beginning of this chapter), are vulnerable to severe infections with the same type of bacteria as the children with agammaglobulinaemia.

Cell-mediated immunity
The thymus is the T cell nursery (see pages 50–51), and children whose thymus has failed to develop (thymic aplasia) therefore lack T cells and they are

vulnerable to a characteristic set of infections. Antibodies are formed more or less as normally, but without T cells from the thymus they cannot make CMI responses. This means great susceptibility to diseases like tuberculosis and measles. The vaccine against tuberculosis (BCG) consists of living but attenuated (weakened) bacteria, and after injection into the arm of a normal person the bacteria multiply locally, stimulating the immune system to make a good CMI response. As a result, the BCG bacteria are eliminated and there is resistance to tuberculosis. But in a child that cannot make that CMI response the normally harmless bacteria multiply in the arm, then spread through the body and eventually cause death. Another disastrous infection in a child with thymic aplasia was measles. Antibody was formed against the invading virus but this was not enough on its own. Without T cells the child could not control the infection and the measles virus multiplied unrestrainedly in the lungs and caused a fatal pneumonia.

Compelling evidence for the role of CMI comes from the modern plague, AIDS. After infection with HIV the body's T helper cells are infected and gradually exhausted or incapacitated (the exact mechanism still poses problems for scientists). The resulting immune weakness comes on slowly, generally over the course of years, and eventually the patient begins to suffer from a characteristic set of infections. Toxoplasma, candida, pneumocystis (see Glossary) and cytomegalovirus are almost universal infections, and these microbes normally remain in the body for long periods (see pages 180–186), but are held in check by CMI (T cell) responses. As the number of T cells falls in an HIV-infected patient, these particular microbes begin to multiply unchecked. They are what cause the disease AIDS. HIV causes the immune deficiency, but the other microbes, now given their chance, cause the actual disease. If it all happened in the first week after infection the disease would have a more dramatic terror.

Very rarely a child is born unable to form either antibodies or CMI. This is called severe combined immunodeficiency (SCID), and such children are exquisitely susceptible to harmless everyday microbes. Some of them have survived after being isolated for a few years inside a microbe-tight container or 'bubble'. In the bubble they are protected from outside invasion, and need only to cope with their own microbes.

Complement

Missing links in the complement system (see Box 7) are uncommon but here, too, there is a clear message about its importance as an antimicrobial defence. Complement makes a big contribution to opsonization and to the killing of microbes (see page 63). Those with defects are susceptible to staphylococci and suffer from repeated infections with gonococci and meningococci, because these are bacteria that are normally killed with this weapon.

Defects in cytokines

Cytokines have been referred to earlier (see Chapter 2). There are so many different cytokines that it is difficult to dissect out their separate roles, and humans do not have naturally occurring deficiences in any single cytokine. But which ones matter most? Luckily that great benefactor of mankind, the laboratory mouse, has been able to answer the question for us. You can produce mice lacking a given cytokine either by interfering with the gene that makes it, or by giving the mouse antibody (monoclonal antibody) against the cytokine to inactivate it. For instance, mice without interferon gamma or without Il-2 (see Glossary) seem normal and healthy, but they develop severe disease if they are infected with herpesviruses or with intracellular bacteria such as *Listeria*. Normal mice successfully control these infections by means of CMI. Evidently interferon gamma and Il-2 form essential links in the chain of a CMI response, and without them the response is crippled. However, one problem with interpreting laboratory studies of this sort has been that when you knock out one cytokine the body can compensate for this by increasing the duties of another cytokine, or increasing the duties of another part of the immune system.

CAN DRUGS STIMULATE THE IMMUNE SYSTEM?

For more than 100 years physicians have been hankering after methods of giving a general boost to the immune system, either to help kill off cancer cells or to treat chronic infections. This is quite distinct from the stimulation of immunity to a specific microbe by means of a vaccine. Many drugs and many treatments have had their vogue, ranging from snake venoms, herbal remedies, and hypnosis, to killed tubercle bacilli and purified cytokines. Several reports show that the BCG vaccine (containing living, non-virulent tubercle bacilli) is effective, not only against tuberculosis but also against certain other infections, presumably because it activates macrophages (see page 64) and thus gives a general stimulus to immunity. But most of the evidence is anecdotal and some of the observations are unconfirmed, so that there are still no widely accepted methods for giving that general boost to immunity. Could it be that some of the reports of success are due to psychological effects (as described under Placebo in the Glossary)?

THE BRAIN SPEAKS TO THE IMMUNE SYSTEM; WHAT HAPPENS DURING STRESS

We know that the nervous system has a say in the regulation of the immune system. For example, major life events such as bankruptcy or grief after death of a spouse have adverse effects on immune responses and make you more vulnerable to infections and cancers. Also you can prevent certain immune reactions in the skin by post-hypnotic suggestion. Many people feel intuitively that the state of mind influences susceptibility to infection. They would maintain that feeling good and feeling happy encourages health, as noted by a silver-tongued writer in Box 9.

The experiment described in Box 10 is an impressive piece of evidence, but it is recent discoveries about actual molecules that have at last given respectability to the idea that the brain interacts with the immune and hormonal systems. We now know that some of the chemical messengers used in the nervous system are also recognized by immune cells. Growth hormone, for instance, is formed by cells in the brain's pituitary gland and also by lymphocytes and macrophages, and many of the cytokines act on brain cells as well as on immune cells. These shared items of language at last provide a chemical basis for the effects of the mind on immunity. Indeed one can look at it this way. Just as the mind has organs (eyes, ears) bringing it information about vision and sound from the outside world, so also it has

---

Box 9 Feeling good

'Health is that which makes your bed easy and your sleep refreshing; that renews your strength with the rising sun and makes you cheerful at the light of another day. 'Tis that which fills up the hollow and uneven places of your carcase, and makes your body plump and comely...

'Tis that which makes fertile, and increaseth the natural endowments of your mind, and preserves them long from decay; makes your wit acute, and your memory retentive...

'Tis that which supports the fragility of a corruptible body and preserves the verdure, vigour and beauty of youth.

'Tis that which makes pleasure to be pleasure and delights delightful; without which you can solace yourself in nothing of terrene fecilities and enjoyments.'

E. Maynwaring (1628–1699)

> **Box 10 Immune depression by the brain!**
>
> Fascinating, if unkind, laboratory experiments tell us that the brain can influence immune events. In 1974, Robert Ader and Nicholas Cohen gave rats water containing saccharin, so that they became addicted to its sweetness. Then, each time the rats drank the sweetened water they injected them with cyclophosphamide, a drug that made them feel sick (and which also depressed their immune system). The rats soon learnt to stop drinking it because it made them feel sick.
>
> So far the experiment is similar to the aversion therapy that was at one time used to cure patients of alcoholism; once the drinking of alcohol has been closely associated with vomiting (caused by an injection of the drug apomorphine) the patient loses interest in it.
>
> At a later stage the rats, when they had partly forgotten their lesson about feeling sick, were reoffered the saccharin-sweetened water. They drank it, but now and quite unexpectedly they began to die of infections and cancer. It turned out that once the sickness caused by the cyclophosphamide had become associated with the taste of saccharin, the saccharin by itself could induce the cyclophosphamide response, *including the immune suppression,* with the resulting infections and cancer. The rats had learnt a conditioned reflex in which the saccharin on its own called into action the cyclophosphamide effect on the immune system. The brain had depressed the immune system.

chemical feelers that keep it in touch with and enable it to influence the workings of the immune system.

We are not surprised to learn that the general state of the body, as well as the mind, influences the immune system. Not only psychological frustration, excessive worry or depression, the sort of events charted on a 'Daily Hassle Scale', but also parachute jumping and exercise, cause changes in circulating immune cells. There is in addition a change in other bodily responses, and wounds, for instance, heal more slowly in people undergoing the stress of caring for elderly demented relatives. The picture is complicated because stressed people tend to drink more, smoke more, sleep less, and are often less likely to consult a doctor. What about physical activity? While moderate exercise increases the number and activity of circulating lymphocytes and polymorphs, the change is in the opposite direction after extreme exertion or overtraining. Theoretically these changes could influence infectious disease (or cancer) but the evidence is not good, and as far as we know moderate exercise doesn't offer the bonus of protection against infection.

At the physiological level there is also a tie-up with hormones. Steroid hormones from our adrenal glands normally enable us to cope with inflammation, injury and infection. During these bodily stresses the brain tells the adrenals to form extra amounts of steroids, which have a beneficial effect by preventing inflammatory and immune damage becoming too widespread (see pages 167-176). You have to produce enough steroid. Patients with diseased adrenal glands cannot respond in this way and may die when infected or injured unless they are given steroids. On the other hand too much steroid can be a disadvantage because it prevents the local inflammatory and immune tissue responses that are essential if infections are to be controlled. Thus, when patients with rheumatoid arthritis are given large doses of steroids to reduce the immune damage taking place in their joints, there is always the danger that chronic infections will light up. We have considered steroids formed during the bodily stresses of inflammation, injury and infection but it is clear that *mental stress* calls forth the same steroid response.

The message from this section of the chapter is that we are at last beginning to understand the interactions between mind and body. Supposing we ask about the possible interactions between mind and mind, the realm of the paranormal. To go into this means taking a great leap into uncharted territory, which seems, by comparison, weighed down with uncertainties, a quagmire of challenges and mysteries.

OUR DEFENCES ARE AFFECTED BY AGE

Hardly any infectious agent causes exactly the same disease in infancy, adult life and old age. There are changes not only in the body's defences but also changes in its reaction to the infection.

Whooping cough is a particularly serious disease in infants and very small children. In 1998 worldwide 346,000 died of it. The reason for this susceptibility is probably that the air channels in the lungs of infants and small children are so narrow that they are easily blocked by sticky mucus. Chest infections tend to be more severe also in old people, and this is partly because their lungs are less elastic and the cough reflex is weaker. Old people, furthermore, are less likely to develop fever and other signs of pneumonia, which can mean a delay in diagnosis and treatment and thus reduced chances of recovery.

Gastroenteritis (diarrhoea and vomiting) takes a great toll of infant life because when the body size is small the loss of water and salts soon becomes life-threatening. This is why *diarrhoea*, caused by a host of infectious agents ranging from viruses to parasitic worms, is a major killer of infants in developing countries, as it was in Europe in earlier centuries. In Asia, Africa and Latin America more than two million infants died of gastroenteritis in 1998, and in a given year a child may spend a total of 60 days with diarrhoea.

Age can affect the severity of an infectious disease because of *changes in the immune response*. Newborn infants are highly susceptible to a great variety of infections, but nature has made arrangements for this. Before birth IgG antibodies from the mother pass across the placenta and protect the fetus. These antibodies last for several months after birth, and should there be an infection during this period, it is milder, and the child gets the opportunity to develop its own immune response. The mother makes a second supreme gift to her child by secreting her IgA antibodies into her milk, which protect the infant against intestinal and respiratory infections. Without this *maternal umbrella*, the infant is much more vulnerable to such infections. As far as infant feeding goes, breast is best.

The illness caused by Epstein–Barr (EB) virus depends on how old you are when you first meet it.

Benjamin, a 17-year-old student, developed a bad sore throat, felt feverish, and went off his food. His throat got better but he felt weak and washed out for the next 6–7 weeks. It wasn't just a cold. His ex-girlfriend had had a similar illness earlier in the year. Benjamin recovered but a month or two later his new girlfriend became unwell, tired, with a sore throat.

The illness was glandular fever, and the virus that causes it (EB virus) is excreted in saliva, not only while you are actually ill, but also for several months afterwards. If you catch it when you are a small child you are hardly aware of it, but if you meet it for the first time in adolescence or adult life you may suffer a fairly long drawn-out illness. Early in life we exchange saliva with our mother and also with other small children. We kiss them, and saliva gets onto our fingers and from there into the mouth. If you put a small amount of a fluorescent dye onto a finger of a 4-year-old boy just as he goes into preschool, the dye can be detected at the end of the morning on the books, tables, chairs, doorknobs, and on the fingers, mouths and faces of all the other children. As we get older our personal hygiene improves and we distribute our saliva around to a lesser extent, so that the next big opportunity for this virus to spread is during sexual kissing, especially 'deep' kissing, which can involve the transfer of a teaspoonful of saliva in a single session. Perfect conditions for the glandular fever virus.

Chinks in the armour; things that go wrong with our defences

If the adolescent missed out on childhood infection he or she is now vulnerable, and is likely to become unwell.

The difference is due to the more vigorous immune response in the older person, nearly all the disease in this infection being caused by the host's own immune response. The cells infected by the virus are B cells and the battle is waged as the T cells recognize the foreign material on them, turn on them, and try to eliminate them. It is an immunological civil war in which lymphoid organs are scenes of frenetic activity (see also page 175). Cytokines are poured out and are probably what make you feel ill.

Various other virus infections (mumps, chickenpox) are milder in childhood, probably for the same reason. In other words, it is best (if there is no vaccine available) to get these common infections over and done with in childhood. Rural areas are less often visited by these infections, so that country people often miss out during childhood. As adults they are then highly susceptible. Mumps, for instance, was one of the commonest causes of sickness in the crowded Allied troops in Europe during WW1. In 1812 it was noted that recruits to Napoleon's army survived longer if they were skinny, ill-fed and came from towns and cities. The larger, muscular, well-fed recruits from the countryside were repeatedly ill with sundry infectious diseases.

Infections that stay around in the body for years in a well-controlled state sometimes light up and cause a fresh episode of disease in old people because of a decline in immune strength. After the age of about 60, people with healed *tuberculosis* sometimes become a danger to others when the bacteria, whiling away the years in some backwater of the immune system, are allowed to become active again. They multiply, spread, and are discharged from the lungs to infect other people. An older schoolteacher who develops a cough may be experiencing a reactivation of old, healed, pulmonary tuberculosis, and can unwittingly infect young children in the class.

Shingles (*zoster*) is a fairly common affliction of old people. After the age of 80, 10% of us suffer from it each year. What happens is that you get chickenpox as a child and recover from it, but the virus then retreats from the immune system by taking up permanent residence in nerve cells in the spinal ganglia, as described on pages 180–186. For some reason the immune response to this particular virus (but not to the related cold sore virus, herpes simplex virus) wanes in old people. The trouble begins because chickenpox virus, lurking in sensory nerve cells, has the habit of reactivating spontaneously. This happens in a single nerve cell somewhere in a ganglion, and in old people the weakened immune response to the virus now allows it to spread to adjacent cells. The disease shingles is the result.

At this stage you may well ask whether there is a general weakening in the immune system as the body ages. This has been a controversial question, and various defects (in T cells, phagocytes) have been reported in the elderly. But the general view is that the immune response of healthy, well-nourished old people is not significantly compromised, and that they cope adequately with other infections. However, a poor diet, especially shortage of protein, zinc and vitamin E, can lead to depressed immunity. Old people may also be more vulnerable because of an age-related deterioration in heart, lungs, or the circulation. Nevertheless, old people enjoy much greater health than they did 50–100 years ago, and their complaints deserve to be investigated and treated like anyone else's complaints, rather than brushed aside as the inevitable burden of 'old age'.

THE SEXUAL PERSPECTIVE ON HOST DEFENCE

Differences between the sexes are generally due to anatomical differences or to the changes taking place during pregnancy, childbirth and lactation. Of those based on anatomical factors the most notable is the shorter urethra in women and its perilous proximity to the anus. Urinary infections (cystitis) are about 14 times commoner in women than in men. Even the mechanical events of sexual intercourse can force bacteria up the urethra so that they become established in the bladder. It makes sense for susceptible women to rinse out the bacteria by passing urine immediately after intercourse.

Pregnant women possess new organs and tissues that offer possible sites for microbial invasion. The placenta is vulnerable to infection by rubella virus or by syphilis bacteria, and these microbes then have access to the fetus. In developed countries congenital syphilis is now rare, but congenital rubella lies in wait if there is a fall off in vaccination against rubella. The drastic hormonal changes of pregnancy have widespread effects. The muscles round the ureter and bladder are relaxed, and because of this the flushing action of urine is less effective, with the same result as in the case of the elderly male with an enlarged prostate gland. Urinary infections are therefore common during pregnancy. Hormonal and metabolic changes also make pregnant women more susceptible to viral hepatitis.

Long ago it was suggested that from an immunological point of view the fetus is a *foreign parasite*, and if this is the case why is it that it is allowed to stay in position rather than be rejected? Is it because the mother's immune response has been suppressed? This has caused much controversy, but it seems unlikely that there are important differences during pregnancy, certainly not the sort that would have an impact on susceptibility to infectious disease. Nature would surely not have allowed this! If there are slight decreases in immune defences the mother compensates by increasing those ancient early defences outlined in Chapter 2. In other words, there must be other more subtle mechanisms, perhaps sophisticated local devices in the placenta, to ensure that the fetus, an immunological foreigner, is not rejected.

THE IMPACT OF HOST GENES ON DEFENCE

Genes seem to affect almost all aspects of life, not only the shape of the nose or the colour of hair, eyes, skin, but even things like temperament or mannerisms. We know that there are genes that control resistance and susceptibility to infectious disease. Consider the *genes for the MHC class 2 molecules*, referred to on pages 53 and 66. Each individual has a slightly different set of them. Because different MHC class 2 molecules present different peptide antigens to T cells or present them with differing efficiency, the response to a given peptide is under genetic control. Clearly a poor immune response to the antigens of a given microbe would mean greater susceptibility to infection with that microbe, although perhaps less susceptibility to damage caused by the immune response (immunopathological damage, see Box 5). Unfortunately there are not many well-documented examples from humans when we consider different individuals. The way MHC differences between different human populations influence infectious disease is described on page 129.

   An impressive example of what are assumed to be genetic differences in susceptibility is provided by the disaster in Lubeck, Germany, in 1926. Instead of the non-virulent bacteria in the tuberculosis vaccine, live and virulent tubercle bacilli were inadvertently given to 249 babies. The dose was identical for each baby but the result covered a wide spectrum. Although there were 76 deaths, the rest of the babies developed only mild illnesses, survived, and were still alive and well 12 years later.

   One of the best ways of checking for genetic influences is to see what happens in *twins*. Identical twins have identical genes, whereas non-identical twins are no more alike than any two brothers or sisters. And one has to focus on twins that have lived apart, not sharing the same exposure to infection. It was not easy to find such a collection of twins, but when it was done the message was clear, and it confirmed the Lubeck story. Eighty-seven per cent of identical twins each had tuberculosis, whereas only 26% of non-identical twins were affected, a striking reflection of the role of genes in this disease.

Sometimes susceptibility to a disease can be taken to the level of a single gene and molecule. This is so in the classical case of *sickle cell anaemia*. Malaria parasites live in red blood cells, feasting on the red oxygen-carrying pigment, haemoglobin. There is a slight alteration in the gene for haemoglobin in people in West Africa and this change, although exceedingly small, means that red blood cells containing the new haemoglobin are resistant to the falciparum type of malaria. This is the most virulent type of malaria, and it is particularly common in this part of Africa. As seen in an artificial environment under the microscope the red blood cells from people with a single dose of the abnormal gene (from just one parent) easily collapse, losing their normal disc-like shape and looking like tiny sickles; hence the name. These people, however, are protected against malaria, a debilitating and often lethal infection. Unfortunately a double dose of the gene (one from each of the parents), although much less common, makes the red blood cells, even when uninfected, so easily damaged and destroyed that the person suffers from anaemia. Yet the advantages of a single dose obviously outweigh the disadvantages of a double dose and the gene persists in the population. See Box 11 for another example of genes, this time MHC genes, linked to resistance to infection.

NUTRITION AND HOST DEFENCE

General shortages

Severe malnutrition interferes with the integrity of the skin and mucous membranes, with the CMI response, and with the activity of phagocytes. But it has been difficult to identify the actual food factors that matter, and to disentangle nutrition from things like overcrowding, poor hygiene and inadequate medical care. This is especially so in the case of tuberculosis. For instance, we are still not sure just why there was a striking rise in tuberculosis in Europe during WW1 and WW2, even in unoccupied countries.

Children with protein deficiency are tragically susceptible to *measles*, and suffer severe skin and corneal lesions, diarrhoea and life-threatening pneumonia. During famines, a quarter to a half of infected children die. Intestinal infections also are often made worse by severe malnutrition, because bacteria then find it easier to cross the intestinal mucosa and invade other parts of the body.

> **Box 11   Psoriasis – the compensations of an unpleasant disease?**
>
> This well-known scaly skin disease is generally a cosmetic handicap rather than a serious threat to health. It affects one in 50 Caucasians, about a third of whom have a first degree relative with the disease. The genes concerned in psoriasis lie amongst those controlling MHC molecules (see pages 53 and 66 and Glossary), which are the ones that also control immune responses. In the affected areas the cells of the epidermis proliferate at ten times the normal rate and are pushed up to the surface and are sloughed off as large scales before they have had time to form a proper outer layer to the skin. T cells have gathered in the affected area, indicating immune activity, and the drugs and other measures used in treatment (such as ultraviolet light) are those that suppress local skin immunity.
>
> Why is it that this disease is so common? On an evolutionary time scale it would seem to be disadvantageous and should have been eliminated. The answer lies in the function of the particular MHC genes associated with psoriasis. It has been suggested that these genes make the T cells react with something in normal skin, which causes psoriasis. But the same response somehow gives resistance to streptococcal infections, so the sufferer enjoys a bonus in the form of protection against scarlet fever and other streptococcal diseases. We know that the T cells in skin lesions of patients with psoriasis show a strong response to streptococci, the bacteria that cause scarlet fever. Moreover a streptococcal throat infection often triggers off the first attack of psoriasis. Until recently scarlet fever and its complications killed many children and it could be that the MHC genes that cause psoriasis were worth keeping because at the same time they gave resistance to life-threatening streptococcal infections.

Shortage of vitamins and other substances

Vitamin A

Vitamin A is needed to keep mucous membranes (especially the conjunctiva and cornea) in good condition. It is probably needed also for making a satisfactory immune response, and the body needs more vitamin A during an infectious disease. Sixty-five years ago a trial was done on 600 English children with measles. In those days measles was sometimes lethal, but those given vitamin A (in the form of cod liver oil) were less likely to die. Now it is abundantly clear that poorly nourished children given extra doses of vitamin A show a dramatic reduction in the severity of measles as well as a reduction in the severity of diarrhoeal diseases.

Vitamin C

Vitamin C deficiency causes the disease scurvy, as Captain Cook discovered in the 18th century when he gave limes to his sailors. The person with scurvy suffers bleeding into the gums, round the hairs in skin, and in muscles. Wounds don't heal and there is anaemia. A French priest who had been in the Crusades described it thus '...the gums and teeth were attacked by a sort of gangrene, and the patient could not eat any more. Then the bones of the leg became horribly black and so, after having suffered continual pain, during which they showed the greatest patience, a large number of Christians went to rest in the bosom of the Lord'.

Increased susceptibility to infection, however, is not a feature of scurvy. For 20 years the Nobel Prize winner Linus Pauling campaigned for massive doses of vitamin C as a remedy for the common cold, although the official view is that most of us get enough vitamin C from our diet, and giving extra amounts serves no useful purpose. The take home message from many studies is that the effect on respiratory infections is minimal, but vitamin C does seem to have an action on polymorph phagocytes. Those who suffer from chronic boils and whose polymorphs are not working normally can be helped by one gram of vitamin C a day.

Vitamin E

This vitamin acts against harmful oxygen radicals (see page 35), and there is little or no evidence that supplements are needed in adults. A 1997 report, however, suggests that it can be important for the immune system, and that elderly people need more than young people. Supplements of 200 mg a day increased elderly people's immune response to various vaccines, as measured by antibody and skin test reactions.

Iron (Fe)

Iron is essential for many bacteria; without it they cannot prosper and multiply. However, in body fluids such as blood and milk the iron is tightly bound to protein molecules, and only restricted amounts are available. Because of this shortage and because bacteria need iron so badly, they make their own set of iron-binding molecules, which enable them to hang on to any iron that comes their way. Many bacteria would grow better in the body if more iron were available. Thus, if large doses of iron are injected into mice to make it freely available, their susceptibility to the bacterium *Pseudomonas aeruginosa* is increased a thousand times.

Oxygen

Oxygen is essential for bacteria such as tubercle bacilli, which also need carbon dioxide (CO_2), both gases being unfortunately available for them in the lungs. Other bacteria, for instance those causing gas gangrene, find oxygen toxic and patients suffering from gas gangrene have been treated by making them breath oxygen under pressure to increase the amount in tissues. The bacteria causing tetanus provide another example, because they grow best when the concentration of oxygen is low. This is why wounds, whether caused by battle injuries or thorns in the finger, are vulnerable to tetanus; they are places where the circulation is interfered with and oxygen is therefore in short supply. Wounds cause trouble especially when they contain thorns and other foreign bodies because these provide nooks and crannies for bacteria to grow in, where they enjoy partial protection from phagocytes. If staphylococci are introduced into the skin on a silken thread, they are 10,000 times more likely to cause a local pus-filled infection than if injected by themselves.

Zinc

Zinc is an essential item in the diet and having too little is harmful to health. Our friend the laboratory mouse shows shrinking of the thymus gland if its diet is deficient in zinc. T cell function and CMI responses are depressed, and also the activity of phagocytes is reduced. In humans there have been many reports on the benefits of zinc supplements to the diet. When infants and small children in Brazil, New Delhi or New Guinea were given zinc supplements to their diet they suffered much less from diarrhoea, respiratory infections and malaria. Middle-aged people given ten times the normal dietary intake of zinc each day show improved T cell function. In another study, sucking zinc gluconate pills at the first sign of a cold greatly reduced the time the cold lasted. Although zinc appears to work on the immune system, this study could indicate that it also has a direct effect on the growth of common cold viruses. But the picture is unclear and we are still undecided whether mild zinc deficiency is common, and whether there is any point in normal people taking supplementary doses of this element.

Selenium

This has received a lot of publicity as an immune enhancer, but here, too, the take home message is unclear.

THE PUZZLE OF POLLUTANTS AND HOST DEFENCE

Cities are places where potentially harmful amounts of chemicals pollute the air, most of them (small particles of black smoke, ozone, sulphur dioxide, oxides of nitrogen) being produced by automobiles. In the choking London fog of 1952 sulphur dioxide levels were five times the WHO recommended maximum, and there were 4000 more deaths due to respiratory illness than would have been expected at that time of the year. But the deaths were in highly susceptible individuals such as the sick, the old, and those with respiratory handicaps. Pollutants are known to have a bad effect on people with chronic bronchitis, and the symptoms from their damaged, permanently infected lungs get worse when sulphur dioxide levels are high. Yet the evidence linking these pollutants with susceptibility to infectious disease is poor, although some of them are known to have an adverse effect on asthma. It could be that in normal individuals the mucociliary cleansing mechanisms can take care of most of the pollutants encountered.

The massive *self-inflicted pollution of cigarette smoking* might well be expected to have a harmful effect on lung defences, because tobacco smoke is known to damage cilia and to load up alveolar macrophages with indigestible debris. There is evidence for this. Respiratory infections tend to be commoner and more troublesome in cigarette smokers, and also commoner in their children, the passive smokers. In a recent (2000) careful study, smokers were four times as likely and passive smokers two-and-a-half times as likely as non-smokers to develop pneumonia caused by that well-known lung invader, the pneumococcus (see Glossary).

One inhaled substance that we are in no doubt about is *silica*, present as a fine dust in mines. Coal miners inhale fine particles of silica over the years, and they eventually develop silicosis. In this disease the lung macrophages that have phagocytosed the indigestible particles of silica are damaged and depleted in numbers. As a consequence the lungs are not protected against tubercle bacilli (see pages 168–172) and there is a great increase in susceptibility to respiratory tuberculosis.

Part 3
THE MICROBE'S RESPONSE TO OUR DEFENCES

Chapter 5

BREACHING THE EARLY DEFENCES

'My home policy; I wage war; my foreign policy; I wage war. All the time I wage war.'
Georges Clemenceau, French politician
(1841–1929).

A MICROBE WITH GOOD ANSWERS

One day at breakfast, when I was five years old, I told my mother that my throat felt sore, and she thought it looked a bit inflamed. But I wasn't unwell, went to school as usual, and that was an end to it. Each week brought the family such a variety of coughs, colds, stomach upsets, cuts and bruises, that this mild sore throat was soon forgotten. It was not until the morning of my 17th birthday, just before the 'A' level exams, that I felt an unfamiliar itching and tingling on one side of the mouth. A day or two later a nasty looking sore appeared there, red and uncomfortable. It scabbed over and healed, but since then I've had several more like it, always somewhere round the mouth. They are cold sores, familiar to many of us, and there is an interesting connection with that childhood episode.

I had been infected with herpes simplex virus, one of the most cunning and ancient invaders of our species. During a playground encounter with another boy who happened to be excreting the virus, a smear of his saliva found its way onto my hand. The virus was soon delivered to a tiny abrasion inside my mouth, entered cells in the vicinity, and began to multiply. First it multiplied in my mouth and throat, which felt sore a few days later, and large amounts of the virus appeared in my saliva, so that I probably infected one or two other children. But I never became ill, and made a good cell-mediated immune response to the virus, eliminating it from this part of the body. I was now immune and it seemed as if the invader had been banished for good.

But no. The virus had entered the ends of the tiny nerve threads that supply sensation to the region of the mouth and then, astonishingly, it travelled up these nerve endings until it reached the nerve cells themselves, seated in the nerve ganglion at the base of the skull. My fine immune response had been powerless to prevent this migration because it all took place inside the actual nerve cell and its endings. The virus now settled down in the sensory nerve cell and made itself at home. It didn't in any way damage the cell. It didn't multiply or release any virus materials (antigens) that might have alerted patrolling T cells and antibodies. It had gone to earth, and as far as the immune system was concerned it was not there. Yet it was securely established in a safe house in my body, just biding its time.

Until that summer day, 12 years later, when something happened. It must have been the strong sunlight on my face the last weekend before the exams when we went sailing in my brother's dingy. I got slightly sunburnt and as the nerve cells of the ganglion received the strong messages from the damaged skin round my mouth things began to happen. In one of the cells the virus came to life after its long sleep. It started to multiply and the infection then spread to a few nearby cells. Stimulated by this activity inside them the nerve cells sent off impulses to the brain, which is what caused the itching sensation round the mouth, although at this stage nothing was happening there. And now the virus set off on another journey, this time down the nerve to the skin around the mouth. It took 2–3 days to reach the skin, at which point the virus left the nerve and set to work infecting all the local cells. By this time the immune system had been alerted and a vigorous response was set in motion. Lymphocytes, macrophages and antibodies poured into the area and together produced the typical inflamed sore. But not before the virus had formed its blister at the skin surface, each drop of the blister fluid containing millions of freshly formed viruses, ready to be carried to anyone who had not yet been infected. The immune defences completed their task satisfactorily and the cold sore healed.

This is the story of cold sores. A sequence of childhood infection, locally controlled by an immune response, but with simultaneous migration of the virus up nerve endings to the sensory ganglion, where the virus takes up residence, safe from immune defences. The stimuli that awaken it so that years later it can re-emerge on the surface of the body, include sunlight, raised body temperature due to other infections, and probably certain types of mental stress.

The sequence (summarized in Figure 18) is the same whatever part of the body the virus enters. If a grandmother has a cold sore and kisses the knee of her young grandson when he runs in crying from the garden after a fall, the virus could enter by way of the scratch on the knee. Now the sensory ganglia down at the base of the spine would be the ones that gave sanctuary to the migrating virus, and the boy's cold sores, if ever he developed them, would be on that knee. Similarly, infection in the genital area means that you would get the painful equivalent of a cold sore in the genital area – genital herpes. Indeed transmission of the virus by this last route has become so common that it has given the genital virus the opportunity to develop its own characteristics, slightly different from that of the regular cold sore. The virologists call this 'below the belt' virus herpes simplex virus type 2, but as you can imagine there are occasions when it can enter ancestral (type 1) territory in the mouth, and vice versa.

Most people have the virus in their ganglia, but we are not sure why only some of us get cold sores. The condition has been recognized for centuries, and it is the only virus infection mentioned by Shakespeare:

> 'O'er ladies'lips, who straight on kisses dream,
> Which oft the angry Mab with blisters plagues'
> *Romeo and Juliet,* Act I, Scene IV

A virus with the ability to re-emerge after many years and transmit the infection again enjoys a great advantage, as set out in Box 31. It explains how the virus manages to maintain itself in small, isolated communities.

We saw in Chapter 4 that once there is something wrong with the natural cleansing mechanisms, or the phagocytes, or the immune defences, a host of otherwise harmless microbes have the opportunity to cause mischief. This is what might be expected. In this part of the book we are concerned with the professionals, the ones that can invade even when the defences are in good working order.

Shrink yourself down to microbial size and consider the daunting task in front of you, as you face the giant with the formidable armour outlined in Part 1. Better still, imagine you are an object the size of a golf ball thinking of invading something the size of a mediaeval castle. The thick walls are well-nigh impregnable unless you are lucky enough to find a damaged area not yet repaired by the army of skilled workers. On the high battlements guards are on the lookout, bristling with crossbows, swords, daggers.

Breaching the early defences

Where the slippery sewers and drainpipes leave the castle, sluice gates open regularly and discharge a torrential flow of unpleasant material. An approach from the air is unwise, to say the least, and inside the chimneys are a formidable array of spikes, grids and sentries. If you do manage to get inside, patrolling guards will see you, raise the alarm, and the tunnels will soon be full of armed soldiers. You are put to death without compunction.

One cannot but admire the successful invader who breaches the defences and then, in the hostile environment of the host, goes on to complete the five obligatory steps (referred to on pages 12–13), which are:

1. Attach to or enter the body (i.e. get round surface defences).

2. Evade the local, the early defences.

3. Multiply.

4. Evade the later, immune defences.

5. Exit from the body.

If the microbe breaches the surface defences, attaches to the body and enters it, it will soon be phagocytosed and killed unless it has some sort of avoidance strategy. Supposing it manages to survive the early defences. Unless it also has an answer to the specific immune defences it will be hunted out, attacked, and destroyed once they come into action.

When we consider the strategies available, it turns out that almost every theoretically possible evasion and avoidance method has been adopted by some microbe or other. You name it, they've done it! Each strategy calls for special molecules, which must be manufactured by the invader, and microbes devote a surprisingly large proportion of their precious genes to this task. Intricate evasion strategies are needed to cope with good defences, and the fact that so much of the microbe's genetic apparatus is spent in this way is an impressive tribute to the power of those defences!

Only a handful of microbes will be referred to in the examples given, but the strategies are in widespread use and have been a recurring theme in the evolution of microbes. Indeed they have helped shape the immune system itself, and have laid down the rules for the battle between parasite and host. Every mutation that helps a microbe in this battle will be retained, and every successful microbe uses one or more of the strategies to be listed. It is their resourceful answer to our defences that enables them to get into the body in the first place, and gives them enough time to multiply and spread so that they can be released and start again in a new host. Some of the viruses are so successful in the evasion business that they stay in the body and enjoy life-long residency. We call these the persistent viruses, and the cold sore example was given at the beginning of this chapter.

As in all military confrontations, a new strategy on one side is met by a counterstrategy on the other. As the host evolves it has been forced to come up with responses to microbial innovations, so it develops more powerful defences and better resistance to infection. Its countermeasures have in turn led to fresh replies from the invaders, and so on, in what amounts to an evolutionary arms race between microbe and host. And because microbes multiply so rapidly and are blessed with a simpler genetic system, they evolve faster and are generally one step ahead. As if to take account of this the host generally has more than one way of carrying out a given defence task. We saw in Part 2 that there are several ways of killing an infected cell, inactivating a microbe, or starting an inflammatory response. This redundancy in the defence system forces the microbe to be even more inventive, because if it gets round any single method of defence it may still be vulnerable to another which operates in a different way.

Let us now set out the strategies used by microbes.

SPECIAL DEVICES FOR ATTACHING TO THE BODY AND ENTERING IT

Whichever surface of the body the microbe first encounters will be well defended, as noted in Chapter 2.

Skin

The superbly constructed barriers of the skin are not easily breached; tightly packed skin scales cover the surface and act as the bricks in the walls of the host citadel. A microbe that colonizes and spends its life on the skin must attach to these skin scales, and should be resistant to dryness, to the fatty acids in skin oils, and to the salty zones round the openings of sweat glands. The resident skin bacterium, *Staphylococcus epidermidis*, fits the bill. It is no accident that this ancient companion of humans adheres to skin scales and resists the saltiness and the dryness of its chosen territory. We all shed a million or so skin scales a day, each one a microscopic raft bearing *S. epidermidis*. The fine white layer picked up when you run a finger along a smooth surface indoors consists almost entirely of shed skin scales. When airborne they spread easily, but under normal circumstances, carrying harmless resident microbes, they cause no trouble. Because the skin is such a good barrier, most microbes only get through at places where there has been a small injury or bite.

Respiratory tract

The air we inhale contains particles. You can see the particles of dust when a shaft of light passes through a dark room. The larger ones (10 microns or so in diameter) settle on the mucous surfaces of the nose, throat and lungs. Microbes are treated like inert particles of dust, and are carried by the ceaseless beat of cilia (up from the lungs, back from the nose) to the throat, where they are swallowed. The microbes that avoid this fate and have an opportunity to start an infection will be those that can stick firmly to the lining cells.

The respiratory pathogens, or at least all those that infect the healthy host, are equipped accordingly. The common cold viruses, influenza viruses and whooping cough bacteria all have special molecules on their surface, each of which fits snugly into sockets present on cells in this part of the body. By these means the microbe sticks to the cell. The same applies to the conjunctiva. If the microbes (chlamydia) that cause conjunctivitis and trachoma (see Glossary) had no way of adhering to conjunctival cells they would be carried away in the tears and lose their chance.

The smallest inhaled particles (less than 5 microns diameter) are often carried right down to the blind alveolar endings of the lungs, where macrophages lie in wait like guard dogs (see Figure 10). The bacteria causing tuberculosis and Legionnaires' disease (see Part 4 and Glossary) start their infection here, and must avoid being taken up and destroyed by alveolar macrophages.

Intestinal tract

The intestine offers a similar choice. Unless the microbe can stick firmly to the wall it will be swept along with the rest of the contents in the inexorable flow to the anus, and will quite probably be killed by acid and bile before it gets there. All the intestinal pathogens have had to respond to this insistent demand for sticking. The gastroenteritis viruses, the bacteria and protozoa causing cholera, typhoid, diarrhoea and dysentery, all carry their special surface molecules, the chemical hooks that allow them to latch onto the wall, resist the onward flow, and stay in one place long enough to start an infection. Tapeworms and hookworms need more substantial anchors, and are equipped with actual hooks and suckers.

The intestine is swarming with resident bacteria, nearly all anaerobes (the type that don't need oxygen), and only 0.1% of them are the traditional *Escherichia coli*. A single bacterium increases its numbers to a hundred million within a day, and the intestines normally contain an unbelievable hundred million million (10^{14}) bacteria, a large proportion of faeces consisting of live and dead bacteria. Multiplication of bacteria is balanced by their continuous passage to the exterior. A faster flow gives less time for growth, and it is interesting that in diarrhoea there are smaller numbers of bacteria in the faeces than normally, although large numbers of the microbe that is causing the diarrhoea. Somehow the residents are tolerated by the immune system, and many of them form substances that inhibit the growth of newcomers, as well as crowding them out.

Urogenital tract

As long as the cleansing mechanisms are intact, the urogenital tract resists all but the specialized invaders, and these must be able to stick firmly to the wall of the vagina or urethra. Only then can they avoid being swept away by urine or fluid secretions. The gonococcus, for instance, has tiny hairs (pili) covering its surface, and on the ends of these hairs are the chemical grappling irons that anchor the bacteria to the cells lining the urethra.

DOING DAMAGE TO THE SURFACE DEFENCES

Some microbes, not content with mere sticking, take a more aggressive, more active approach to surface defences. For instance, whooping cough bacteria (*Bordetella pertussis*) and the bacteria once thought to cause influenza (*Haemophilus influenzae*) both release substances that either damage cilia or slow their beat. Therefore the mucociliary escalator described in Chapter 2 doesn't sweep the bacteria away so effectively and they have a better chance of starting an infection. Cholera bacteria (*Vibrio cholerae*) wriggle about in the intestinal mucus and also release a substance that liquifies this mucus, thus increasing the chance of making contact with an epithelial cell. Amoebae are notoriously mobile, and those responsible for amoebic dysentery (see Glossary) move about in the intestine until they find host cells to attach to. They feed on bacteria and on debris discarded from host cells, but can also phagocytose and kill these cells. The resulting damage and inflammation causes ulcers in the intestine. Sometimes, and for unknown reasons, the amoebae become much more aggressive and they burrow deeper into the wall of the intestine and can reach the liver.

You can get leptospirosis or schistosomiasis (see Glossary) if your bare skin is immersed in infected water, because these microbes actively penetrate the skin, as mentioned earlier.

COPING WITH THE PHYSICAL ENVIRONMENT

Successful microbes must also adapt to the physical environment at body surfaces, which is often unsuitable or hostile. The survival strategy for *S. epidermidis* on the skin has been mentioned. Microbes like polioviruses that enter and leave the body via the intestine, tend to resist the acid conditions and the bile that they will encounter on their journeys. This is not as simple a task as it sounds, and only some of the intestinal pathogens are resistant. Cholera bacteria (*V. cholerae*) resemble most bacteria in being quite sensitive to acid. A normal person must drink a hundred million of them (easily acquired from faecally contaminated sources) if an infection is to be started, but when the acid in the stomach is first neutralized by swallowing some bicarbonate of soda, a mere thousand bacteria are sufficient. *Helicobacter pylori* adopts a more direct method for coping with stomach acid, as explained in Box 12.

GETTING ENOUGH FOOD

All parasites take their food from the host; otherwise they cannot grow and multiply. Most food items are only too readily available, but iron is an exception. It is a vital item and getting enough can be a problem. Almost all (99.9%) of it is locked up inside red blood cells and the rest is almost as inaccessible because it is tightly joined to proteins present in blood and milk. Indeed, it looks as if the host has deliberately made it hard for microbes to get their iron. In response, as might be expected, many microbes have iron-hungry molecules that suck the iron away from the host, sticking to it even more firmly than do the host proteins, and so ensuring that they get enough of this essential element.

COPING WITH INTERFERONS AND COMPLEMENT

Interferons

The interferon defence is switched on very early after infection and poses a serious threat to invaders, especially viruses, as described in Part 2. It would be a useful strategy either to resist the action of interferons or to prevent them being formed.

It has not been easy to get convincing evidence that interferons really matter in host defence. Enormous amounts of purified interferon have to

---

Box 12 The acid connection of Helicobacter pylori

Helicobacter pylori is the helical bacterium of the pylorus, and the pylorus
is the end of the stomach that opens into the intestine, acting as the gate
leading to the intestine (Greek, *pyloros* = gate-keeper). This bacterium,
discovered only 15 years ago, is present in more than half of people over
the age of 50, and there are at least a hundred million bacteria per
person. It attaches to the stomach wall and causes inflammation,
dyspepsia, and in some people a duodenal or gastric ulcer. For this reason
ulcers are now treated with antibiotics rather than just with antacids. The
bacterium protects itself from stomach acid by releasing an enzyme
(urease) that manufactures a tiny cloud of ammonia around it, locally
neutralizing the acid. This is its strategy.

H. pylori spreads from person to person by the faecal–oral route, and it
is one of those microbes whose impact has been altered by modern
hygiene. Until the 19th century nearly all humans carried the bacteria as
part of the normal flora. Today you are likely to be infected as a child if
you live in a developing country, whereas in industrialized countries, with
improved hygiene and less crowding, the bacteria spread less readily
through the community and infection is generally put off until later in
life. The effect of age on the infection is uncertain, and we still have a lot
to learn about *H. pylori.*

The bacteria generally stay in the stomach for years, and seem to cause
ulcers by increasing the amount of acid produced. Why is it that only
some of those who are infected get ulcers? Perhaps it depends on the
strain of bacteria. Psychological stress certainly encourages ulcers, and
probably another factor is smoking.

The idea that *H. pylori* causes duodenal ulcers was demonstrated when a
courageous doctor in Perth, Western Australia, drank a potion containing
the bacteria and developed an ulcer. Not only gastric (stomach) ulcers but
also, later in life, stomach cancer, is associated with *H. pylori* infection.

---

be dribbled into the nose of volunteers to make any impact on a common
cold-type virus infection. But the fact that viruses go to a great deal of
trouble to avoid interferons can be taken as a testimony to their value. For
instance, adenoviruses (see Glossary) have a special gene for blocking their
action, and without this gene the amount of viral multiplication in cells is
reduced ten times.

Interferons exert their protective action after becoming attached to host cells. They fit into the socket of a special interferon-receiving molecule present on the cell surface. Poxviruses (see Glossary) have adopted a cunning strategy by forming their own interferon-receiving molecules which are released from the infected cell. These mop up the interferon before it can stick to nearby host cells, which therefore remain unprotected.

Other viruses such as hepatitis B have ways of preventing interferons being formed in the first place. In animals there are several virus infections that stay in the body for life with complete failure of the host to produce interferons. These include lymphocytic choriomeningitis (LCM) virus (see pages 159–160 and Glossary) in the perpetually helpful mouse. Interferon works against LCM virus and it would be nice to know why it is not produced and why this defence has therefore failed.

Complement

Complement counts as part of the early defence network because its complex cascade of reactions can be triggered off without the need for antibody (see Box 7). It is also part of the immune network and often co-operates with antibody. It is no accident that many microbes, such as *T. cruzi* (see Glossary), herpes simplex and Epstein–Barr (EB) virus, either avoid lighting the complement fuse, or produce substances that interfere with the body's control of complement. It is not clear exactly how they manage to do this, but it enables them to reduce local inflammation and prevents white blood cells arriving on the scene.

Upsetting suicide

This is as good a place as any to remind you that when a virus gets into a cell, the cell, for the benefit of the whole body, often chooses suicide rather than staying on as a virus factory. A noble gesture, and a good defence strategy, as shown by the fact that many viruses (hepatitis B, adenoviruses, EB virus) have found that it pays to interfere with the cell's suicide (apoptosis) programme.

OUTMANOEUVRING THE PHAGOCYTE

Consider a microbial invader the size of a mouse confronted with a well-equipped killing machine the size of a battleship. Is there any escape? How can the invader avoid those weapons and stay alive?

A microbe that is easily recognized, ingested, and killed by phagocytes is by definition unsuccessful – it is doomed. The successful ones have tackled this particular problem and have in some way or other learnt how to interfere with or avoid the phagocyte. The contest between the two has been proceeding for many hundreds of millions of years, and if there are possible ways round the phagocyte problem then some microbes will have discovered them. The possible strategies, which are easiest to understand if you refer back to Figure 8, are as follows.

The microbe kills the phagocyte

This is the most straightforward thing to do, possible in spite of the small size on the invader. It can be accomplished by releasing a toxin that either damages the cell wall of the phagocyte, or damages the wall of its lysosomes (see page 36 and Glossary). Lysosomes are packets of powerful enzymes and one of the toxins formed by streptococci causes the lysosomes of polymorphs to explode and liberate their damaging contents into the cytoplasm, as a result of which the cell dies. The toxin has made the lysosomes act as 'suicide bags'. Staphylococci produce a substance called leucotoxin, meaning white cell toxin with a similar action. Sometimes the microbe releases the toxin after it has been phagocytosed and is inside the cell. This is the way macrophages are killed by the *Shigella* bacteria responsible for food poisoning. The macrophages can be said to have died of food poisoning!

The microbe prevents chemotaxis

As an example of this, the main bacterial culprit in periodontal disease (see page 138) inhibits the movement of phagocytes into the infected pockets between the gums and the teeth. Also, substances that kill the phagocyte, such as the streptolysin toxin, often prevent it moving about (in other words prevent chemotaxis) when present in lower concentrations. They can also prevent phagocytosis itself (see below), because this too entails movement. A paralysed phagocyte is as good as dead, from the microbe's point of view.

The microbe prevents phagocytosis

A phagocyte that has been damaged or paralysed by the microbe poses no threat. Otherwise, to avoid being phagocytosed the microbe needs to have a surface that is not recognized by the phagocyte as foreign, or a surface which makes the act of phagocytosis difficult. Classic surface substances acting like this are the slimy polysaccharide capsule that coats the pneumococcus (see Glossary and Chapter 3), and other substances on streptococci. You can watch under a microscope as a phagocyte tries to engulf one of these bacteria blessed with a protective layer of slime round it. It is like trying to pick up a wet fish. The phagocyte advances, arms outstretched for the embrace, but the bacterium slips away from its grasp. Many other microbes foil the phagocyte in this way.

Once the host has produced antibody the tables are turned. The antibody, often with the help of complement, acts as an opsonin and thus makes things easy for the phagocyte, as described in Chapter 3. Occasionally the host is lucky enough to be able to opsonize the microbe before antibody has been formed. This is done by depositing complement directly onto the microbe, using the so-called 'alternate pathway' (see Box 7). Microbes, however, have devised their own ingenious answers to opsonins. It would have been difficult to think up the following strategy from first principles, but it is used so frequently that it must be very effective. Although strictly speaking it prevents opsonization by interfering with the action of antibodies (immune defences) it is mentioned here because of its impact on phagocytosis.

Staphylococcus aureus (the golden staph) has on its surface a substance called *Protein A*, which binds tightly to the stem on the Y of antibody molecules (see page 56). As a result, each bacterium gets covered with as many as 100,000 molecules of whatever antibody is in the vicinity, and of course hardly any of them will be directed against the bacteria. Any that are capable of reacting with the bacteria cannot in any case do so because they are anchored in a useless upside-down position, the portions that combine with antigen (the ends of the Y) waving freely from the surface. An opsonic effect is now out of the question because phagocytes only recognize the stem of the antibody, not the antigen-combining arms that are now offered to them. Protein A is not the only one that does this. Similar proteins adorn the surface of streptococci, herpes simplex (cold sores), varicella zoster (chickenpox) and cytomegalovirus.

Virulent staphylococci have an interesting alternative strategy. They release an enzyme (coagulase) that forms a coagulated network of host material (fibrin) round them and on their surface, which makes it difficult for phagocytes to get near them.

The microbe gets taken up into the phagocyte but resists being killed

If the microbe accepts phagocytosis yet is able to survive, even to multiply in the phagocyte, it is in a strong position. The phagocyte that cannot kill will end up packed with living invaders and unable to control the infection. Moreover, if it is still mobile and not sick it can carry the microbe round the body and perhaps at a later stage allow it to enter a distant organ. This is a feature of many virus infections. Measles, mumps, and others get a free ride round the body, safe inside migrating macrophages, and this enables them to invade the respiratory tract (measles) or the salivary glands (mumps).

There are four ways a microbe can avoid being killed in the phagocyte. If you look at Figure 8 and imagine yourself as a microbe trapped in a phagocyte's death chamber (vacuole), you will see that these are the logical alternatives.

A. Stop the lysosomes discharging their lethal contents into the phagocytic vacuole

After virulent tuberculosis bacteria have been phagocytosed they liberate a special substance that stops the lysosomes in their tracks and prevents them coming to the vacuole and fusing with it. You can see them lined up round the vacuole, keeping their distance, unable to proceed further. The microbes causing Legionnaires' disease (see page 212), toxoplasmosis and cytomegalovirus (see Glossary) act in a similar way. Unfortunately for the microbe there are other killing methods that do not depend on fusion of the lysosomes.

B. Resist the killing process in the phagocytic vacuole

Staying in the killing chamber of the phagocyte means death for most microbes. Yet some of them have learnt how to resist killing, and even survive and to multiply. These include *Listeria* (see Glossary), and the bacteria causing the plague (*Yersinia pestis*) and tuberculosis. We do not understand how they do it. Is it merely a matter of having a good coat of armour? It is not enough to have rather indigestible walls, as in the case of tuberculosis, because killing takes place before digestion. Preventing acidification of the vacuole would be more useful, and there are microbes that manage to do this. It was especially bad news for phagocytes when a few microbes such as *Leishmania* and Q fever (see Glossary) learnt how to survive and multiply even when surrounded by acid. Learnt to do it so well in the case of Q fever that now it will not grow without the acid!

A few bacteria (gonococci, staphylococci) possess an enzyme called catalase that looks as if it could actively interfere with lysosomal weapons. Hydrogen peroxide is an integral part of the killing system (see Figure 8), and catalase eliminates hydrogen peroxide by converting it into carbon dioxide and water. If any of these bacteria fail to produce the catalase or produce less of it, they are killed more easily in polymorph phagocytes.

Some microbes achieve the ultimate insult to the phagocyte by not only resisting being killed and multiplying, but also by having special structures that force the phagocyte to supply them with nutrients. *Toxoplasma* (see Glossary) and *Legionella* build conveyer belts round themselves, by way of which the phagocyte delivers food parcels and energy.

C. Escape from the phagocytic vacuole

An early escape from the phagocytic vacuole could mean an escape from death, but how can this be accomplished? Viruses have come up with an interesting method. Many of them (such as influenza) use this method firstly to get into the cell. The virus is surrounded by a membranous envelope studded with a special protein and it is this protein that attaches to the outer membrane of the host cell. The virus and the cell membranes then fuse, allowing the contents of the virus to be discharged free into the cytoplasm of the cell (Figure 13). This is how the virus gets in, and it can now begin to multiply. If the virus has been phagocytosed, then because the phagocyte's vacuole is lined with a similar membrane, fusion can also take place with the wall of the vacuole. If the phagocyte is the cell in which the virus is destined to multiply, as with HIV or dengue virus (see Glossary), escaping early from the vacuole is a distinct advantage. One or two bacteria, such as *Shigella* and *Listeria*, resort to a more aggressive method. As soon as they have been ingested they destroy the wall of the vacuole.

D. Don't enter the phagocytic vacuole in the first place – enter the cell by some other method

It is not easy to avoid death once you are in the phagocyte's vacuole, and an alternative, for those that have chosen to grow in this type of cell, is to enter by some other method. Virulent *Shigella* and *Salmonella* practice active penetration, boring their way in at the cell surface without being taken up into a vacuole. Some (toxoplasma, trypanosomes, dysentery amoebae) have special enzymes that punch entry holes in the cell wall. As mentioned above, many viruses get into the cell by fusing their outer coats directly with the cell surface (Figure 13), thus avoiding the phagocytic vacuole.

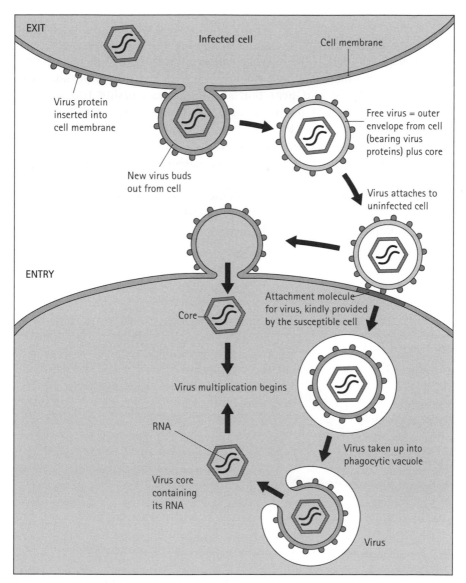

Figure 13 Intimate invaders – how viruses like HIV and influenza get into and out of cells. The virus *exits* from the cell *above* by a 'budding process', so that the outer coat (envelope) of the fully formed virus contains cell membrane plus virus proteins. This way the cell suffers little damage, but some viruses (e.g. polio) get out by disrupting and destroying the infected cell. The newly formed virus can now *enter* (infect) the cell *below* (a) by fusing directly with the surface of the cell or (b) being phagocytosed and then fusing with the wall of the phagocytic vacuole. *Attachment molecule for virus, kindly provided by the susceptible cell.

Breaching the early defences

It is when the microbe has already been coated with antibody that the phagocyte sticks firmly to it, engulfs it, and the killing process is triggered off (see pages 60–62). If the microbe can avoid setting off this trigger or if it can get in by some other pathway it will have a less stormy passage. You will not be surprised to hear that the microbes causing tuberculosis, Legionnaires' disease, whooping cough, listeriosis and leishmaniasis either interfere with the action of the trigger or have special molecules that (when not coated with antibdy) can stick them to a different part of the phagocytic cell, away from the dangerous parts that stick to the stem of the antibody molecule.

Luckily for the host the above strategies are usually foiled once enough antibody has been formed to cover the microbe. It is then fully opsonized and is successfully taken up and killed.

Chapter 6

HOW TO EVADE IMMUNE DEFENCES

'Such as do build their faith upon
The holy text of pike and gun;
Decide all controversies by
Infallible artillery;
And prove their doctrine orthodox
By apostolic blows and knocks.'
from *Hudibras*
by Samuel Butler (1612–1680).

The very existence of successful infectious agents tells us that host defences do not form an impenetrable barrier. They doubtless deter many potential invaders, but infections are nevertheless common. More than 400 different microbes infect humans and 150 of them quite frequently. Many owe their success to interference with the immune defences. They do this so often, and in so many different ways, that the rest of this chapter will be devoted to the subject. We will begin with the story of a well-known immune evader.

The master chameleon makes fun of the immune system

The great 19th century explorers of Africa, including Livingstone, Stanley, Speke and Burton, encountered a veritable hail of infections carried by biting insects and contaminated food and water. Dysentery, malaria and other fevers were added to the physical dangers of the expeditions.

David Livingstone (1813–1873) was a physician, explorer and missionary (although he himself only converted one African). He carried out three pioneering expeditions in Africa, discovered the Victoria Falls, helped expose the cruelties of the slave trade and clarified the geography of the almost unknown interior of the continent. During the first expedition (1854–1857) he suffered no less than 27 attacks of fever, was laid low with dysentery, and would have been susceptible to the trypanosome parasites causing sleeping sickness. On the title page of *Missionary Travels and Researches in South Africa,* his 1857 book describing this expedition, there is an engraving of the tsetse fly, which transmits sleeping sickness.

His third and last expedition began in 1865. He set out to find the source of the Nile and it was on this expedition that he was 'found' by Stanley ('Dr Livingstone, I presume') after being lost to the world for five years. Later, tired and ill with dysentery, when milk alone would have restored his health and strength, his six cows were attacked by tsetse flies and died soon after. The dysentery continued and he got thinner and weaker. Perhaps he was never actually infected with the trypanosome parasites, but being deprived of that milk made him an indirect victim of the tsetse fly. In the last entry in his journal on April 27, 1874. he wrote: 'Knocked up quite and remain...recover...sent to buy milch goats'. His antibodies, lymphocytes, phagocytes and other defences had been doing their best under an appalling load of microbial invasion plus physical and nutritional stress. Exhausted and weak, he died on May 1.

The sleeping sickness parasite (trypanosome) infects the salivary glands of the tsetse fly. This fly is a large daytime feeder, very persistent, able to bite through a cotton shirt, and it transmits the infection to cattle and antelopes as well as humans. The parasite enters the body when the fly bites, grows to form a local swelling in the skin, and invades the blood. The person becomes ill with fever, but subdues the infection by forming antibodies. The resourceful parasite now changes the molecules of its outer coat so that the antibodies no longer react with it, and it then starts multiplying again. The sufferer makes another set of antibodies, but the parasite responds with a further change. This can go on for months. Each time the immune response catches up with the parasite by forming antibody, it alters its coat. The waves of infection continue until either the parasite is eliminated or, more commonly, the host dies.

The disease becomes serious when the parasites in the blood invade the brain, causing mental disturbances, somnolence (hence 'sleeping sickness'), coma, and death. In 1803 Thomas M. Winterbottom, a physician who practiced in Africa for four years, described the disease in African slaves: '...the patient gradually wastes away. The disposition to sleep is so strong, as scarcely to leave a sufficient respite for the taking of food; even the repeated application of a whip, a remedy that has been frequently used, is hardly sufficient to keep the poor wretch awake...the disease usually proves fatal within three or four months.'

Trypanosomes have genes for about 100 different surface molecules (antigens), which are switched around during the infection. One in ten of its genes are devoted to this, and it is a strategy that has paid off, enabling this chameleon-like parasite to run rings round, almost make fun of, the immune system. The full name of the African form is *Trypanosoma brucei*. Sir William Bruce (1855–1931) was a military physician, born in Melbourne, Australia, who discovered Malta fever (brucellosis) in Malta, and in Africa showed that the tsetse fly carried sleeping sickness.

The specific immune defences come into operation after about a week. As described in Part 2, they consist of antibody and cell-mediated arms, each co-operating with complement and with phagocytes. The evasion story is the same as with phagocytes. If there are ways round the defences, then microbes will have discovered them. Indeed if there is a possible microbial strategy that does not appear to have been used, then closer investigation may show that it has in fact been used, or that the strategy has defects that we had not appreciated. We can go further than this with viruses, because it looks as if some of the larger ones (poxviruses, herpesviruses) have genes whose function is unknown because they interfere with types of host defence that have not yet been discovered. In other words, successful microbes know more about immunity than do the immunologists!

Viruses are in a special category. Most types of microbe cannot help advertising their presence. They make a noise, chemically speaking, releasing toxins and other molecules that act as alarm signals for the host and cause inflammation. Invading viruses are different. They release no toxic chemicals, conserving their more modest number of genes for essential tasks once they are inside the host cell. If they infect cells without damaging them they can stay in the body for weeks, silently entering the blood and distant organs, unnoticed by the host.

The persistent viruses, the ones that stay in the body for years or throughout life, have been the most successful evaders of immune defences, and they will be mentioned as examples with monotonous regularity. These immunological acrobats can make the immune defences look silly and almost silence them. A more modest evasion of immunity can also be useful. Any virus that takes more than a week or so to spread through the body and do its business will benefit if during this period it can temporarily hold off and interfere with immune defences. In humans this includes measles, mumps, rubella (German measles), chickenpox, and many others. The original virulent strain of virus causing myxomatosis in rabbits (see Box 2) produces at least five different substances that interfere with the immune system, and when this virus is genetically engineered so as to be incapable of forming any one of these substances it is much less virulent.

A DOZEN DEVIOUS DEVICES

Although we will now look at a dozen ingenious strategies in immune evasion and salute the extraordinary resourcefulness of microbes, we nevertheless have to acknowledge that the immune response generally does a good job. All but the most cunning invaders are eliminated.

One method of evading the immune system is by carrying out a very brief raid, a hit and run infection, that is all over before immune defences have been mobilized and come into action. As far as the eleven other methods go, invading microbes, especially the viruses, can be thought of as *spies that have entered a foreign country*. Their strategies are exactly comparable to those of a successful spy. As might be expected, the persistent microbes turn out to be the most resourceful, but others benefit from a few extra days in which to accomplish their mission in the host, and have found these strategies worthwhile.

1. Cause a rapid 'hit and run' infection – the commando raid

This is the strategy of 'Get it over with quickly, before immunity comes into action.' In military terms it is a commando raid, completed before the main defences have been mobilized. Because, at the first encounter, the immune response takes a week or so to get under way, a fast moving microbe has the opportunity to complete the infectious process without exposing itself to immune defences. Speed is esssential. If it can infect, multiply, and be shed to the outside world in less than a week it does not have to worry too much about immunity. It must attach to the body surface, must face up to early and local defences, but when it is quick it avoids the strongest defence of all.

The infections that come into this category are those that remain on the body surfaces, which include (Figure 5) the respiratory, intestinal and urogenital tracts as well as the skin. After initial attachment the microbe spreads over the surface layer and multiplies without penetrating deeper, until enough offspring have been formed to ensure transfer to a new host. The immune response does, of course, unfold, and is often the force that finally terminates the infection, while the antibodies and memory cells formed make the individual resistant to another infection with the same microbe. But this all happens too late to stop the invader doing what it wanted to do.

On the respiratory surfaces, the success of the hit and run strategy is indicated by the great wealth of viruses that use it. Humans are hosts to about 90 different common cold viruses, and 20–30 different influenza and other respiratory viruses.

In the intestinal tract the viruses and bacteria responsible for diarrhoea and dysentery do the same thing. It is all over within a few days. In the urethra, the bacteria causing gonorrhoea and other types of urethritis multiply and are released, uncomfortably and in large numbers, within a week.

2. Stay indoors – don't show your face at windows

When using this strategy the microbe, if it grows in cells, stays there and doesn't betray its presence by releasing recognizable foreign materials (antigens). The cell is its sanctuary, and the immune system does not know it is there. Both the cold sore virus described at the beginning of this chapter and the chickenpox/shingles virus (see Part 4) stay in sensory nerve cells for years in this way. The virus lies low, not forming antigens or offspring until the need arises. Even when these particular viruses do multiply, they are fortunate in being able to spread directly from cell to cell without venturing into the dangerous extracellular world.

The bacteria that live inside cells (leprosy, *Listeria*, *Brucella*) must come to terms with the cells' own defences but sheltered in the cell they at least enjoy some protection from immune forces. Malaria parasites have their headquarters in liver cells, where they are safe from immune attack. They expose themselves, unavoidably, when they sally forth into the blood to invade red blood cells.

3. Interfere with the immunological informers (the MHC) that might betray your presence

As explained in Box 8, the powerful cytotoxic (killer) T cells only act after they have recognized a foreign protein fragment (peptide) displayed on the surface of the infected cell and held in the arms of the host's own MHC molecules. Without the MHC part of it the cytotoxic T cell does not respond.

It fails to release its cytokines and is unable to kill the infected cell. In other words the MHC molecule acts as an immunological informer.

Many persistent viruses have discovered methods for interfering with MHC display on infected cells. HIV, cytomegalovirus, herpes simplex virus and adenoviruses (see Glossary) prevent MHC getting to the cell surface. The mechanisms are now understood in fascinating detail at the molecular level. It is a brilliant microbial strategy but the host, in the eternal ding-dong battle with the invader, has been able to come up with an answer. The task of the cytotoxic T cell, which can no longer recognize the infected cell, is handed over to another type of T cell, the *NK (natural killer) cell*. This recognizes precisely those cells that *don't* have the MHC label, assumes they are infected, and kills them!

And then, as another example of the sequence of strategy and counter-strategy, there is cytomegalovirus, an old hand at immune evasion. Cytomegalovirus has answered the threat of the NK cell by forming its own fake MHC molecule. The fake MHC is no good for the delicate task of holding peptides in position, yet the NK cell thinks it is host MHC and doesn't respond to the cell that carries it. It therefore passes by, leaving the cell to the tender mercies of cytomegalovirus.

4. Find a safe place to stay

At the body surface it is harder to call into action all the defences available deeper inside the host. IgA antibodies are eventually secreted onto these surfaces, and certain antimicrobial substances are available, but under normal circumstances the defences present in the blood, including IgG and IgM antibodies, complement, immune cells and phagocytes are in short supply. Without a good deal of inflammation and leakage of these weapons from local blood vessels the host cannot bring all the troops onto the battlefield. This makes things easier for the hit and run surface invaders described above. It also means that these body surfaces are attractive sites for permanent residents, especially for the persistent viruses.

The skin surface is inhabited by resident bacteria and by the wart viruses. There are more than 70 different types of wart virus, adapted to life in different parts of the body, ancient companions of human beings. A wonderful adaptation to their chosen site gives them almost total indifference to immune responses, as shown in Figure 14 and described in Box 24. Another possibility is to invade the dead outer layers of the skin, or the dead cells that form hair and nails (see Box 13).

Box 13 Fungal focus on the dead

The dead outer layers of the skin, or the dead cells forming hairs and nails, seem ideal sites for microbes that do not need living cells, because they are well beyond the reach of immune defences. The microbes that have taken advantage of this are certain specialized *fungi*. They love the keratin in dead cells. Each species favours a certain part of the body, and several of them gain access to humans from cats, dogs, and even hedgehogs. The fungus grows and stays in place because skin is always renewing itself and nails and hairs lengthen, so that fresh supplies of dead cells with their cargo of keratin are always arriving.

The fungus has to be careful. If it grows down too fast it will encounter host defences, and if it doesn't grow fast enough it will be shed from the body and separated from its host. Not an easy life. A trickle of antigens from the fungus enter the body, and cell-mediated immunity (CMI) and antibody are formed. When the antibodies react with fungal antigen present in the skin it results in inflammation with redness and itching, but the parasite is unaffected. In the old days the red, rounded, scaly skin areas, and the bald patches where infected hairs have dropped off, were thought to be due to worms. Hence the use of the word 'ringworm' and the Latin word 'tinea', a maggot or grub. The types of fungus adapted to the skin itself prefer moist areas such as between the toes (athlete's foot) or in the groin (jock itch or tinea cruris), although in warm, humid countries like Papua New Guinea the general body surface is just as hospitable. Treatment can be difficult, and for antifungal drugs to reach infected nails and hair they need to be taken by mouth; it often takes a long time.

Glands often provide a safe refuge. The cells lining the tiny tubules in the kidney harbour the polyoma viruses (see Glossary) and those lining the ducts of the salivary gland harbour glandular fever (Epstein–Barr, or EB) virus and other herpesviruses (Figure 14). These tubules and ducts carry urine and saliva to the exterior, and the lining cells are inside the body but face the outside world. The viruses are in a quiet backwater where, tucked away from police surveillance in the form of T cells and serum antibodies, they will not be disturbed.

The *brain* is another place where investigating T cells and antibodies are infrequent visitors, and here, as long as there are no local disturbances

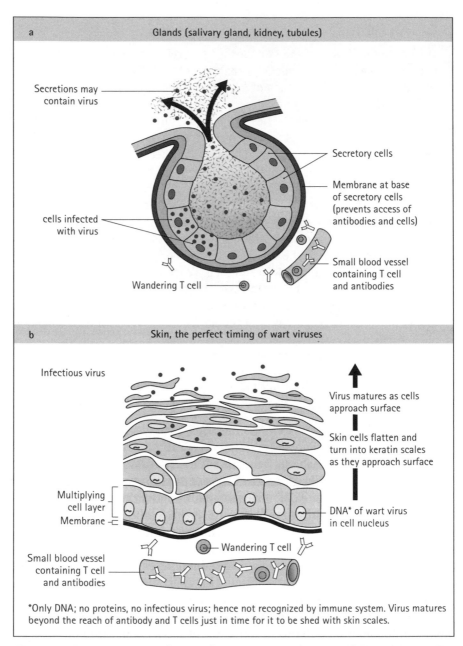

a — Glands (salivary gland, kidney, tubules)

Secretions may contain virus

Secretory cells

Membrane at base of secretory cells (prevents access of antibodies and cells)

cells infected with virus

Small blood vessel containing T cell and antibodies

Wandering T cell

b — Skin, the perfect timing of wart viruses

Infectious virus

Virus matures as cells approach surface

Skin cells flatten and turn into keratin scales as they approach surface

Multiplying cell layer
Membrane

DNA* of wart virus in cell nucleus

Small blood vessel containing T cell and antibodies

Wandering T cell

*Only DNA; no proteins, no infectious virus; hence not recognized by immune system. Virus matures beyond the reach of antibody and T cells just in time for it to be shed with skin scales.

Figure 14 Safe hiding places. A) Glands (salivary gland, kidney, tubules). The secretory cells in glands are like skin cells insofar as they face the outerworld and are normally out of the reach of blood antibodies and T cells. B) Skin. The perfect timing of wart viruses.

(inflammation), a microbe can sometimes enjoy a quiet life. But it is not a common hiding place. Alarms are easily set off, and in the brain almost any infection gives acute and dramatic results. Bacterial meningitis and viral poliomyelitis are life-threatening, crippling, examples.

Hence the microbes that achieve long-term residence in the brain have done so by treading very gently and slowly. They are all viruses, as might be expected in view of a virus' ability to replicate in a subdued, almost silent fashion. Before the measles virus vaccine was widely available, an occasional child who seemed to have recovered from measles and eliminated the virus, would 'overlook' and leave behind a few infected cells in the brain. The virus then began to multiply exceedingly slowly, spreading from one brain cell to another, and finally, 5-10 years later, it had done enough damage to cause encephalitis. Until then the child had been perfectly well, but now began to suffer from a serious and ultimately lethal disease. All this was of no value to the original infecting measles virus because it provided no outlet to the outside world. The disease (the tongue-twisting 'subacute sclerosing panencephalitis' or SSPE) was no more than an unusual, unnecessary, and unfortunate illustration of the versatility of measles virus.

5. If possible dress like a native

It goes without saying that a spy cannot afford to be conspicuous, and certain microbes have taken this on board as a strategy.

Wear the real native clothes
One way of self-concealment is to take up host molecules to cover the microbe surface. Worms such as the blood-fluke *Schistosoma* provide the nicest examples of this sort of immunological disguise. The schistosome covers itself with various substances (immunoglobulins, MHC molecules, glycolipids) present in the blood of the host, so that antibodies and T cells assume that it is not a foreign object, fail to recognize it, and leave it alone.

Make your own native clothes
Alternatively the microbe could possess molecules of its own that were modelled to look like host molecules, thus baffling the immune policemen. This is referred to as 'molecular mimicry' (see Box 14), and there are many examples of it. The trouble is, we are not sure just how useful it is to the invader.

Box 14 Imitating the host

About 20 years ago scientists got excited about molecular mimicry when their studies showed that it was a very common thing. Using a computer they tested protein molecules from different viruses and searched for similarities to protein molecules present in normal humans. They found that the proteins of many viruses had small fragments (peptides) that were strikingly similar to those on human molecules such as myelin basic protein, a component of the insulating layer round nerve fibres. Presumably the findings would be much the same if microbes other than viruses were tested.

Is this a molecular accident or can it be regarded as a microbial strategy? It seems that when very small peptides (up to six amino acids long) are similar it may be nothing more than an accident. In the case of a larger peptide (7–8 amino acids) the similarity could be because this segment carries out the same essential molecular task in both microbe and host rather than because the microbe is trying to imitate the host. It looks as if we have to be cautious when we talk about the meaning of these similarities.

One consequence of molecular mimicry is that the host immune system, which often identifies such molecules in spite of the resemblance to 'self', sometimes makes a response that also reacts against host materials. An autoimmune reaction has been generated. For instance, the person suffering from glandular fever (EB virus infection) makes antibodies to red blood cells. These antibodies are useful to the physician because they provide a blood test for glandular fever. If they are present they can be demonstrated by their reaction in the test tube with red blood cells. Likewise in syphilis, it has long been known that antibodies to certain components of syphilis bacteria also react (cross-react) with normal body components, and this provides us with the original, classic diagnostic test, the Wasserman reaction. If the patient has antibodies to extracts of normal heart it means that he has syphilis, because these are the antibodies that also react with materials from syphilis bacteria.

Unfortunately immune responses directed against the microbe do occasionally damage the host, as explained in Box 5. In the disease rheumatic fever, a person infected with a certain type of streptococcus makes antibodies to the bacteria that react also with his own heart, and he develops myocarditis (inflammation of the heart). Autoimmune reactions triggered off by microbes are thought to play an important part in diseases such as multiple sclerosis and rheumatoid arthritis.

6. Keep changing your appearances

Spies who keep changing their appearance certainly make things harder for the police. If you are a microbe you can evade immune defences, however powerful and irresistible, by constantly changing your antigens. This is a widespread practice.

Changing antigens as the microbe spreads in the community
Changing antigens is easiest at the level of the whole population of susceptible individuals. Many 'hit and run' microbes constantly change their antigens (by mutation) as they circulate through the host community, forming new variants or strains. If the antigens of a new strain are sufficiently different, then this strain will not be recognized by individuals with immune memory cells for the original strain, and it can reinfect them. This encourages the appearance of new antigenic variants, and therefore they are always arising. Some of the new strains will be able to infect the same set of hosts and spread once again through the community, and in this way the microbe evolves.

The dozens of different strains of streptococci (*Streptococcus pyogenes*) have arisen partly by this process, and they can therefore give you many attacks of rheumatic fever (see above and Glossary) which, if not prevented by penicillin, eventually causes permanent heart damage. One of the reasons people can suffer more than one attack of gonorrhoea (in 18th century London the writer Boswell recorded 19 episodes in entertaining detail!) is the existence of many antigenic variants. Immunity to one doesn't protect you against the others.

Antigenic variation is a major feature among the respiratory and intestinal viruses. The 100 or so different common cold viruses, the influenza viruses (see Box 15), and many of the different intestinal viruses or 'enteroviruses' probably arose as antigenic variants.

Other microbes, however, show little or no antigenic variation. This is especially so for those that do not cause 'hit and run' infection of body surfaces, but instead spread through the body and infect different organs. Measles, mumps and tuberculosis stay much the same over the years and throughout the world. Minor changes can be detected between the different strains, but once you have developed immunity to any one of them you are protected against the disease. Two and a half thousand years ago Hippocrates gave us an unmistakable description of mumps, and it would be fascinating to see whether mumps virus from this era is the same as it is today. All that is needed is a time machine!

Box 15 Influenza virus keeps one step ahead

Influenza virus is the classic example of antigenic variation. As it spreads through the community there are small changes in its surface proteins due to mutations. These accumulate, until strains emerge that are new enough, different enough, to start another journey through the same susceptible population. This population was infected with the original strain and developed immunity to it, but the new strain is different enough, antigenically speaking, to reinfect them, and it has thereby evaded the immune defences. Influenza epidemics occur locally, and at any time many different strains are in circulation. It is a gradual process, and the phenomenon is called *antigenic drift*.

Very rarely something else happens and a completely new type of influenza virus appears quite suddenly. What takes place is that two different viruses, one from birds and the other from humans, accidentally get into the same cell. A very unusual event, but it might occur, for instance, when a person living close to birds (possibly ducks in Southeast Asia) is infected with a human and with a bird virus at the same time. A hybrid virus emerges, with new antigens not previously encountered by humans, and this virus can now spread through the entire population of the world. This is how pandemic influenza arises; outbreaks were charted in 1889, 1918, 1946, 1957 (Asian flu) and 1968 (Hong Kong flu). Are we due for a new one? (see Part 5). These sudden and dramatic changes in influenza virus are due to what is called antigenic *shift* as contrasted with the small, slowly accumulating changes of antigenic drift.

Changing antigens during infection of a given individual

A less common, but in some ways more interesting type of antigenic variation is that which occurs during a single infection of a single individual. The disease *relapsing fever* is caused by a bacterium (*Borrelia recurrentis*) transmitted to humans by the bite of an infected body louse. It occurs in Africa and in South America, and caused 50,000 deaths in North Africa and Europe during WW2. A week or so after infection antibodies are formed, killing the bacteria and removing them from the blood. The fever subsides. But new strains of bacteria with different surface antigens then arise, so that a week later bacteria reappear in the blood and cause a fresh episode of fever. This in turn is terminated by the appearance of a fresh set of antibodies. The process continues, with as many as ten episodes before the patient completely recovers. Hence the name relapsing fever. The bacteria present a moving target to the immune system, evading it by changing the antigenic goalposts, and thus prolong their stay in the patient and increase the chance of infecting more body lice and more people.

Sleeping sickness is a disease in Africa caused by parasitic protozoa (try-panosomes), and these play a similar game of hide and seek with the immune system, as described at the beginning of this chapter.

Among the viruses there are only one or two that go in for this sort of antigenic variation within a given host individual. A patient infected with *HIV* may harbour several different strains of virus, and a different set of cytotoxic T cells needs to be generated to deal with each strain as it appears. This perhaps helps this successful virus to stay put in the host, and it certainly makes vaccines a difficult problem.

7. Interfere with police communication

Just as with the police network, communication and collaboration between immune cells (policemen) is the foundation for an effective response. Cells must talk to each other, and this ensures that the response begins, develops, and terminates in a co-ordinated fashion. In the immune system communication depends on intimate physical contact between cells, and the language is the local release of different chemical messengers or cytokines, as outlined in Part 2. The cytokine network is complex, and immune cells bear special molecules to which the different cytokines attach and can then deliver their message.

An attractive looking microbial strategy would be to interfere with the signaling system between immune cells, so that a properly co-ordinated response to the infection was impossible. This strategy has indeed been adopted, and many instances have come to light recently. So far, most of the examples are from viruses. Scientists have identified virus molecules that are similar in their structure either to the host's cytokines or to the molecule on the cell surface to which the cytokine attaches. For instance, the virus causing glandular fever (EB virus) produces a substance with an extraordinary resemblance to an important cytokine called interleukin-10. Interleukin-10 interacts with other cytokines, has effects on immune cells, and it pushes the response in the direction of antibody rather than CMI (see Figure 11). The fake interleukin-10 produced by EB virus and released by infected immune B cells has the same actions, and its sudden appearance in inappropriate amounts in the midst of other immune cells upsets the normal regulation of the response. The emphasis now is on antibodies, useless against this virus, rather than on effective CMI, which is all to the advantage of the invader. It is another example of molecular mimicry.

The poxviruses produce an impressive assortment of molecules that imitate cytokines. They also produce some equally disruptive ones that imitate the molecules on cells to which cytokines attach, and therefore mop up locally formed cytokines. The immune system has a hard time with viruses like these. What better, more subtle, way to upset the response.

8. Take the bull by the horns and invade police headquarters (the immune system)

This is the most logical, the most audacious strategy. To put it another way, if you want to overcome them, attack them; *if you want to evade, then invade*. It is surely no accident that so many microbes, especially the ones that persist in the body, infect immune cells. Once again, viruses offer the best examples.

Almost every persistent virus infects either B cells, T cells, macrophages or dendritic cells (see Glossary). This can disrupt the immune response in several ways.

- First, by actually killing off immune cells.

- Second, by altering immune cells so that they cannot carry out their job. Viruses often infect cells without killing them, and can upset specialized functions of the cell such as the secretion of hormones or cytokines.

- Third, by liberating large amounts of viral antigens in the vicinity of immune cells. Appearance of large amounts of antigen in immune tissues has a disruptive effect because the amounts in these tissues are normally carefully controlled. T and B cells can be completely switched off or 'tolerized' if exposed to large amounts of antigen. Instead of being stimulated they now fail to respond.

During the response to an infection the T and the B cells that react with the invader's antigens are in a state of intense activity, and dividing rapidly to increase their numbers. It so happens that certain viruses are especially partial to these activated, dividing cells, and readily infect them. If these particular cells are then killed or otherwise put out of action, it amounts to a neat removal of just the cells that might otherwise have terminated the infection. HIV parasitizes the immune system. It infects and probably kills T helper cells, especially the ones that are activated and dividing in response to the infection, and the final decline in their number in the blood heralds the onset of those other infections characteristic of AIDS.

Compared with HIV glandular fever (EB) virus has adapted in a more sensible way to a life in the immune system. Most of us are unwitting hosts to this quieter, less damaging parasite (see pages 81–82, Chapter 4). It infects B cells, activates them, and makes them produce whatever antibody they were destined to produce. As a result a whole series of irrelevant antibodies appear, probably upsetting the immune response to EB virus itself. Loyal T cells, however, eventually gain control by killing off most of the infected B cells. But a small number of B cells (about one in a million) remain infected and stay in the body, probably for life. Some are present in bone marrow, ready to give trouble if given to an uninfected individual in a bone marrow transplant.

Another highly successful parasite of the immune system is cytomegalovirus, which infects macrophages once they have been activated, and interferes with immune responses. There are many other examples, such as measles, mumps, rubella and adenoviruses, each of which infects T or B cells.

Microbes invading the immune system generally depress immune responses

From the point of view of a given microbe the thing to aim for is to prevent the immune responses to itself. Although it would be nice if the immunosuppression was precisely targeted against only the antigens of the invader, it usually affects the response to a wide range of antigens. Thus, on the day a child develops the brilliant rash of measles, the immune skin reaction to tuberculosis and other antigens is depressed, and remains so for several weeks. This sort of thing happens in a very large number of virus infections. But it is gentle and temporary.

The virtues of moderation

It makes sense that the microbe should achieve its purpose without overstepping the mark. A certain amount of damage to the host may be unavoidable, such as the diarrhoea or respiratory discharges needed for transmission of intestinal and respiratory infections, but too much damage or unnecessary damage will in the end reduce the number of host individuals available to the microbe. This is also true for immunosuppression. HIV infection follows the virus tradition in interfering with host immune responses, but the immunosuppression is long-term and ultimately devastating. This virus has gone too far. Instead of the moderate and temporary effect engineered by other human viruses, it runs amok. With shortsighted indiscretion, HIV proceeds to destroy the immune system, and in the end its host.

It is interesting to note that microbes tend to overstep the mark when they infect a species, which is a dead end as far as transmission goes. Because they are not transmitted any further this type of host is irrelevant for the microbe's future. From this point of view it doesn't matter if the host suffers severe disease. A host of human infections come into this category, including rabies, Lassa fever, Legionnaires' disease, psittacosis (parrot disease), brucellosis, leptospirosis and the dreaded Ebola and Marburg virus infections (see Part 4 and Glossary). None of them is transmitted effectively from person to person, and humans are unnecessary for their survival. From the point of view of these microbes, human infection and damage is an unfortunate but irrelevant accident.

HIV arose from similar viruses infecting primates in Africa, and it is only within the last 30–40 years that it has developed the capacity to be transmitted regularly between humans. It looks as if it has not yet had time to settle down to a less damaging and ultimately more successful life in our species.

9. Create a diversion

Strictly speaking this strategy is appropriate for a true invader rather than a spy. Set the alarm bells ringing, call out the police, create a diversion, while you proceed unobtrusively with your business. One way microbes can achieve this is by causing a general switching on of B cells and T cells. Instead of stimulating just those cells that respond to the microbes' antigens a vast range of B and T cells, of all sorts of reactivities, are affected and begin to divide. It is called 'polyclonal activation'.

When B cells are switched on in this way a wide spectrum of antibodies are produced, and this is what happens in EB virus infection (see above), in chronic malaria (in which only a small proportion of the vast amounts of antibody formed is directed against the malaria parasite), in syphilis, and in trypanosomiasis (sleeping sickness).

Other microbes cause a general switching on of T cells throughout the body. They do it by liberating molecules of something called 'superantigen'. A regular antigen stimulates only the very small proportion of T cells that react specifically with it, perhaps 1 in 100,000, as described in Part 2, but a superantigen fires off as many as a tenth of all T cells, whatever their reactivity. They respond, dividing and releasing cytokines in a disruptive, unco-ordinated fashion. In the midst of this immunological chaos the microbe goes about its business.

Highly potent superantigens are formed by several common bacteria, including *Staphylococcus aureus* and *S. pyogenes*. The superantigens of *S. aureus* originally made their name as the toxins responsible for staphylococcal food poisoning and the scalded skin disease seen in small babies (see Part 4). There seems no reason for the bacteria to produce toxins that do such things, but the superantigen action looks very much like the basically useful one that helps in the eternal battle with host defences.

10. Have something ready up your sleeve in case of local encounters with police

Under this heading I want to tell you about methods for interfering with immune responses locally, anywhere in the body. Some of them have been referred to earlier. If the response has already begun and T cells and antibodies are in the neighbourhood, searching out the intruder with murderous intent, it is worth having a few last minute tricks. One of these is to deposit a fog of host protein round yourself. This is what *S. aureus* does, thanks to the enzyme coagulase, as described earlier in this chapter. Cells and antibodies cannot make their way through this fog, and the bacteria are protected.

When humans, sheep or goats are infected by the dog tapeworm, the parasite ends up in the liver or lungs and is enclosed in a thick wall. This is called a hydatid cyst, and its thick impenetrable wall gives long-term protection from antibodies and immune cells.

A more aggressive last minute local device would be to secrete a substance that actually destroyed antibodies (or complement). Sure enough, the gonococcus and a few bacteria infecting the respiratory tract (*Haemophilus influenzae*, pneumococci) secrete an enzyme that breaks up the IgA antibodies that the host delivers to mucosal surfaces.

11. Bribery

Does a microbe ever give its host a present in return for residency or a safe passage though the body? This would amount to symbiosis.

The resident bacteria inhabiting the skin receive food, shelter, and are tolerated immunologically, in return for a few small gifts to the host. They metabolize secretions from sweat and sebaceous glands to form odoriferous substances that have a social and sexual function, in non-human animals at any rate. They probably also give protection against colonization of the skin with pathogenic microbes. Resident bacteria in the intestine, too, protect against harmful microbes. In many herbivorous animals the intestinal residents are not only useful but essential for life, and the fermentation chambers in the intestines of cows and rabbits are described on page 8, Chapter 1.

The above examples of bribery are of resident, non-invasive microbes. The possibility that this strategy could apply to a microbe that invaded the body was until recently no more than an interesting possibility. Who else but a mouse could hand us a nice example? (See Box 16.)

12. Get the police to make the wrong sort of response

It would make a spy's job easier if the police could be persuaded to monitor all radio, e-mail and internet transmissions without checking the letters or newspaper ads through which the spy actually communicated. In terms of a microbe getting round immune defences it means engineering a type of response that sounds good but doesn't work against the invader.

It looks as if microbes use this strategy. We have seen in Chapter 3 that if an immune response against a microbe is to be successful it must have the appropriate balance between antibody and cell-mediated responses. For instance, antibodies are of little help against tuberculosis; good CMI responses are needed to fight this invader. On the other hand, CMI responses are no good for poliomyelitis virus, which is susceptible to antibodies.

Could a microbe 'decide' to induce one type of response (antibody or CMI) rather than the other, 'decide' to induce the type of immune response that was ineffective? Would a microbial variant that called forth the non-protective type of response be selected out and replace the others? Surely yes, and we have seen (see page 121) how the herpesvirus (EB virus) causing glandular fever forms its own imitation (interleukin-10-like) cytokine that pushes the host response towards an ineffective antibody response rather than an effective CMI response!

It would also help a spy if he were assigned to a country with an inefficient police force, poorly trained in identifying spies. In terms of the invading microbe this means that things will be easier if the host is

---

Box 16   Bribery by a breast cancer virus

Mice are commonly infected with mouse mammary tumour virus, which can cause breast cancer. It stays in the body for life, because the mouse fails to make an effective immune response to it. The virus is shed into milk and this is the main way it is transferred from mother to infant. When the virus first enters the body it infects B cells, but it can multiply only to a limited extent in these cells. To complete its destiny and spread to other mice it needs to reach the mammary glands and before it can do this it must undergo further multiplication. Only then will there be enough virus to invade the blood and undertake the journey to the mammary gland. The problem is solved by increasing the local supply of B cells. The virus forms a superantigen type of molecule (see above) which causes B cells to divide. After growing in the new supply of B cells there is enough virus to be launched into the blood on a successful journey to the mammary gland target. When scientists removed the superantigen from the virus it could no longer be transmitted from mother to infant.

So where does the bribery come in? It turns out that this particular superantigen plays an important part in the mouse's immune system. Indeed, it was identified by immunologists as an interesting molecule long before the discovery that it was formed by this virus. Mouse mammary tumour virus, therefore, can be said to bribe the mouse with a useful molecule in return for board and lodging and a local supply of the cells it needs to grow in.

The discovery of this virus in 1933 stimulated an excited search for an equivalent breast cancer virus in humans, but none was found.

Bribery sounds such a good idea for a virus that it is surprising there are no human examples. A herpesvirus bribery fantasy is described in the last paragraph of Chapter 11.

---

constitutionally incapable of making a strong immune response to it. Does this happen? As we saw in Part 2, the host's immune capacity is controlled by numerous genes, such as those responsible for the MHC molecules. Everyone has a slightly different set of these genes, and individuals (or species) with a poor (narrow) selection will be able to present, on their antigen-presenting cells, a more limited range of antigens. This means they will have a more limited range of responsiveness to microbial antigens, which

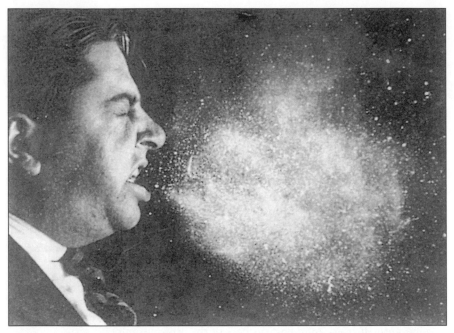

Figure 15 Droplet dispersal following a violent sneeze. Most of the 20,000 particles are seen coming from the mouth. (Courtesy of the American Association for the Advancement of Science.)

may lead to difficulty in controlling certain infections. It is best to have a broad spectrum of possible responses to cope with the vast antigenic range of the potential pathogens (see Box 17).

In a person suffering from the lepromatous type of leprosy (see also Part 4) the nasal mucosa and the skin are teeming with leprosy bacilli because of a failure in the CMI response. There are plenty of antibodies, but they are no good against leprosy bacilli. Macrophages are in the infected areas but they have not been turned on by T cells as described in Part 2 and are useless for phagocytosing and killing the invader. The bacteria of leprosy do well in this type of person, who has the MHC molecules that go with poor CMI response to leprosy. Compare this with the patient suffering from the tuberculoid type of leprosy. Here, due to an excellent CMI response, macrophages are loaded with bacilli, killing them and keeping the infection under control. Unfortunately some of the leprosy bacteria have got into sensory nerves, and the immune attack against them damages these nerves, causing loss of sensation and eventually the onset of disfiguring changes in hands and feet.

> **Box 17 Cheetahs and humans**
>
> The story from cheetahs suggests that having a wide range of MHC molecules matters at the level of the species. These animals have an unusually restricted range of MHC molecules, and this goes with great susceptibility to a variety of infections. Cheetahs suffer from devastating epidemics. The story, it seems, can be extended to humans. As outlined in Chapter 5, the inhabitants of isolated areas of the world have proved highly susceptible to introduced infections that were new to them. We now know that their MHC is far less varied than that of the teeming populations of Europe, East Asia and sub-Saharan Africa. Evidently in these major continents the greater variation in MHC molecules, resulting in a wider spectrum of immune responsiveness, meant that there were always a few individuals who could handle any new infections and hand on this gift to their offspring. Among the more isolated communities, in contrast, this sort of evolutionary pressure to keep the MHC molecules as varied as possible was less prominent, and they paid the penalty.
>
> Individual hosts with genes that confer a poorly protective response to an invading microbe will tend to disappear. Therefore, as with other aspects of the microbe–host confrontation, an evolutionary balance is to be expected, with the microbe often one step ahead. Microbes always tend to be changing their antigens, and if they hit on one that the host responds poorly to, the new strain of microbe that possesses it will be more successful. As long as it doesn't do too much damage to the host species, it will replace the other strains. It is perhaps going too far to look upon this as a microbial strategy, but the sequence of events seems a logical one.

ARRANGING FOR EXIT

The subject of exit and transmission to fresh hosts does not strictly come under the heading of 'Evading immune defences'. It is included here because microbes have mechanisms for arranging for it or encouraging it. The subject of transmission, moreover, is poorly understood, as has been illustrated by the things people want to know about HIV and AIDS. Can you get it from a mosquito bite, from oral sex, from a shared toothbrush, from the communion cup? Evidently the parasites, but not the research workers, have been engrossed in the business of spread.

The host does not live forever, and no infectious agent can survive unless it is transferred to fresh hosts. This transfer generally takes place from one of the body surfaces (see Figure 5), and is arranged by the microbe in the sense that it has to arrive at the exit site in large enough numbers and, if necessary, become cast off into the environment.

Respiratory infections

Respiratory infections are spread by droplets, and it pays microbes to stimulate the cough or the sneeze reflex. The common cold viruses induce a flow of virus-laden fluid, and whooping cough bacteria provoke a sticky mucus and make you cough. After a paroxysm of coughing the child, out of breath, sucks in air and makes a characteristic whooping noise.

During a good sneeze tens of thousands of droplets are dispersed from the nose and mouth (Figure 15). The largest (>1 mm diameter) soon fall to the ground and would only infect someone else by direct face-to-face contact, but the smallest particles (1–4 micrometres diameter) stay suspended indefinitely in the air. Water evaporates from the droplet but as long as the microbe is not killed by drying you can be infected if you come into the room at a later time.

Droplets are formed in smaller numbers during talking, and this is a source of infection during face-to-face contact. During singing, much larger quantities are formed, and it is dangerous to sing in a choir with people suffering from respiratory tuberculosis. Microbes, however, are not known to induce talking or singing – rather the reverse. More droplets are formed when the consonants f, p, t and s are used, and the fact that (in the English language, at least) many of the most abusive words begin with these letters is surely not without significance. A spray of droplets, potentially infectious, is delivered with the abuse.

Intestinal infections

It pays these microbes to induce diarrhoea because diarrhoea is such a wonderful material for contaminating the environment and spreading the infection to others. Microbes that infect by way of the intestine are shed by the same route. Some of them, such as hepatitis A virus, grow in the liver and get back into the intestine by entering the bile channels. It is not surprising that successful intestinal microbes tend to be resistant to bile as well as to stomach acid and digestive enzymes.

Saliva

Many microbes are shed into saliva, and often (e.g. mumps) grow in salivary glands. Transmission via saliva is especially prominent in young children, as described on page 93, Chapter 4. If a child going to preschool has a small amount of a fluorescent dye applied to one finger, then at the end of the morning the dye is on the mouths, fingers and bottoms of most of the other children, as well as on the toys, door handles, chairs and tables. The lifestyle of the herpesviruses (see also pages 180–187, Chapter 8) makes use of this 'salivary promiscuity'.

Mucosal infections

This includes infections spread by kissing and by sexual intercourse, and actual contact between mucosal surfaces is generally needed. Although microbes must arrive on the relevant mucosal surfaces, they are not known to have a say in transmission to other people by increasing mucosal contacts. But come to think of it, it is a microbial strategy that *could* be useful. Supposing a person with a salivary or sexually transmitted type of infection felt more affectionate, more amorous, due to a substance formed by the microbe. This would give that microbe such a headstart over the others that it would replace them. Perhaps suitable substances with this aphrodisiac type of action are non-existent and unattainable, whether by microbes or by diligently searching humans.

Skin contact

Here, too, the microbe must be present in the right place at the right time, but, apart from the timing of the maturation of wart viruses (see pages 116 and 157–159), there are no special adaptations.

Blood transmission

Transmission by biting insects or ticks is one of the most ancient of methods. The microbe has to be present in the blood in large enough amounts and at the right time to infect the bloodsucker, as outlined in Box 1 for certain parasitic worms. Are there any other adaptations? It has been argued that when you are sick you are more likely to be bitten by mosquitoes. You lie still and pay less attention to such nuisances. But it is going too far to elevate this to the status of an actual microbial strategy. Most infections are transmitted best if the host feels well enough to move about in the community rather than retire to bed.

Certain blood infections, such as hepatitis C and hepatitis B viruses, are transmitted by contaminated needles, syringes and blood transfusions, and sometimes there seems no other significant route of transmission. Obviously this could not have been the case more than a hundred years ago, before the modern era of needles and syringes. In the old days the needles for acupuncture, tattooing and ear-piercing were surely not used often enough to be reliable methods for the regular spread of infection. As an alternative there is the possibility that these infections were originally spread by biting insects or ticks!

Worldwide about 12,000 million injections are given each year, about one in ten of them for vaccines. In parts of Southeast Asia and Africa disposable syringes are often used more than once ('if it still works, use it again') without being properly sterilized in between. The WHO is encouraging the use of new 'autodestruct' syringes where you can't withdraw the plunger once it has been pushed in. Fountain pen-sized jet injectors that do the job without needles may also help with this problem.

Some parasites alter their host's behaviour so as to increase the likelihood of transmission

In the types of animal that keep rabies going (dogs, foxes, wolves) the virus invades the brain and alters behaviour so that the infected animal is more likely to bite another individual and spread the infection, as described on pages 148–149, Chapter 7. Other examples include certain parasitic worms that infect land-living insects. For the next stage in its life cycle the worm needs to enter water, in which it can mate and lay its eggs. Accordingly, several of these worms alter the behaviour of the parasitized insect, making it throw itself into water.

Part 4
THE DISEASE

Chapter 7

FROM RESIDENTS TO BIG KILLERS

'From winter, plague, and pestilence, good lord, deliver us'
from *Summer's Last Will and Testament*
by Thomas Nashe (1567–1601).

UNEXPECTED INTRUDERS ROUND THE EYES

Pull out one of your eyelashes and examine the base of it under a strong hand lens or, better, under a microscope. As likely as not you will see something to astonish you. There, attached to the base of the lash, is a tiny, spindle-shaped creature, a third of a millimetre long, whose eight stumpy legs are slowly moving! It is the hair follicle mite (*Demodex folliculorum*), and it lives down in the hair follicle or in a sebaceous gland, sucking the juices from local cells. Most of us, whatever our race or country, have these parasites. They are the commonest 'outside' parasites (ectoparasites) of humans.

The female lays her eggs down in the follicle and about 10 days later, after going through larval stages, the adult mite emerges onto the skin surface and begins the perilous search for a fresh, unoccupied follicle. In most people the mites do no harm, and the wonder of it is that we can have parasites as large and accessible as this without being aware of their existence.

What about those powerful host defences that took up so much space in earlier chapters? Have they failed again, allowing this mite to live so commonly, if unobtrusively, in those little pits in our skin? Immune responses doubtless take place, but this ancient, well-adapted parasite evidently has the right answers. There are 65 different species of *Demodex*, each one adapted to a different animal host. Generally they give no trouble, but those in dogs, cattle and goats can cause mange, and people occasionally develop blepharitis (redness and itching of the eyelids), curable by antiparasitic ointments.

THE RESIDENTS

Some microbes have established themselves as permanent, more or less harmless, residents

Before looking at the diseases caused by microbes we must remember the normal residents. After describing such an array of powerful defences it is embarrassing to contemplate the vast numbers of microbes that make us their permanent home. Most of them are like the eyelash residents described above and do no harm.

We are born germ-free, but during that dangerous descent through the vagina to the outside world we pick up local residents, and the first crying gasp introduces other microbes into the throat and lungs. Over the course of the next few weeks our body is dramatically colonized by an army of specialized microbes. These come mostly from our mother, are referred to as the *normal microbial flora*, and have been the close and constant companions of our species for millions of years. Adam had 'em. Why do we call them a 'flora'? They are not flowers, although when you examine them under high magnification they can resemble an area of dense forest, a pile of apples, sometimes branches swaying in an aquatic current. Perhaps the best explanation, without stretching the etymology too far, is that they can be said to flower or flourish in their chosen habitat.

The *skin* houses altogether about 10^{12} bacteria, of 5–6 different types. The *lungs* are normally sterile, but the *nose, mouth, teeth, throat* and also the *genital mucosa* and *intestine* are home to a variety of resident microbes, specially adapted to life at these sites (Figure 16).

The mouth is densely settled with 10^{10} bacteria of more than 20 different types, attached to cheek, tongue, teeth and throat, and it is a good place to be, rich in food particles and nourishing debris from local cells (see Box 18).

Urine as it leaves the bladder is normally sterile, but on the way out it picks up resident bacteria living just inside the urethra, and these have to be taken into account when urine is tested from patients with cystitis.

In the vagina the resident lactobacilli (as many as ten million per drop of vaginal secretion) produce acid and tend to keep out other microbes (see pages 29–30).

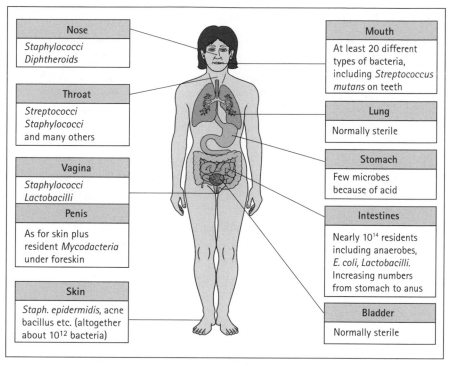

Nose
Staphylococci *Diphtheroids*

Throat
Streptococci *Staphylococci* and many others

Vagina
Staphylococci *Lactobacilli*

Penis
As for skin plus resident *Mycodacteria* under foreskin

Skin
Staph. epidermidis, acne bacillus etc. (altogether about 10^{12} bacteria)

Mouth
At least 20 different types of bacteria, including *Streptococcus mutans* on teeth

Lung
Normally sterile

Stomach
Few microbes because of acid

Intestines
Nearly 10^{14} residents including anaerobes, *E. coli, Lactobacilli.* Increasing numbers from stomach to anus

Bladder
Normally sterile

Figure 16 The residents – the normal microbial flora.

The *intestine* is teeming with nearly 10^{14} residents; compare this with 10^{13}, the total number of cells in the body! The intestinal residents are in a state of flux, influenced by age, diet, hygiene and hormones (the role of hormones in acne was described in Chapter 1). The intestinal flora of breast-fed infants is simpler and gives greater protection than does the flora of bottle fed infants, and vegetarians have a different intestinal flora from meat eaters. A balance is maintained, and individuals differ. Indeed if we think of it literally as a flora, each of us cultivates a characteristic garden in our mouth and intestines.

There are only a few residents in the stomach because of the acid but the numbers increase from then on until in the large bowel, the main growth area, there are 10^{10} (ten thousand million) per gram of contents. Most people think of *Escherichia coli* (see Glossary) as the predominant bacteria but they are present only in modest numbers, and they consume what little oxygen is available. The vast majority is anaerobic bacteria that either don't need oxygen or are actually poisoned by it. The large bowel is a seething

---

Box 18 Animalcules in the mouth

The richness of microbial life in the mouth was first described by the Dutch naturalist Anthony van Leeuwenhoek (1632–1723), 200 years before the time of the great microbe hunters Louis Pasteur and Robert Koch. Leeuwenhoek was a cloth merchant whose hobby was making magnifying lenses, and he constructed a simple microscope with a magnification of up to 200 times, grinding the lens himself. One day in 1683 he took a tiny fragment of the whitish matter from between his teeth, mixed it with water, and placed it on a piece of glass under his microscope. He saw 'with considerable wonder, that...there were many very little living animalcules, very prettily amoving...another sort went so nimbly and hovered so together that you might imagine them to be a big swarm of gnats or flies, flying in and out among one another.' He drew them and it is clear that they were bacteria, including spiral-shaped ones (spirochaetes) and rounded ones (cocci), which are common between the teeth and gums. In what appears to be the first-ever experiment in antisepsis he '...put a little wine-vinegar to this stuff mixed with water; whereupon the animalcules fell dead forthwith.'

Unfortunately the space between the teeth and gums has no natural cleansing mechanism, and the food debris that accumulates here is best removed by mechanical means (the toothbrush or dental floss). When the resident bacteria in the plaque on the teeth overstep the mark and colonize the space under the gums they cause inflammation and an influx of polymorphs. The inflamed gum (gingivitis) bleeds easily and the substances formed by the multiplying bacteria cause bad breath. If the inflammation goes further (periodontitis) the structures that support the teeth are weakened, a pocket develops between the gum and the teeth, and the teeth become loose. In the UK one in five adults has chronic periodontitis. The painful holes in teeth (caries) caused by the resident *Streptococcus mutans* in dental plaque were described on pages 4–5 of Chapter 1.

---

cauldron of microbial activity, producing a multitude of substances (see Box 19), and bacteria normally comprise about a quarter of the total faecal mass. Three things make the intestines the body's largest battlefield. First its sheer size as an organ, second the massive load of resident microbes that have to be kept under control, and third the constant threat of invasion by this route (see pages 150, 163–165). There is in fact in normal people a continuous passage of exceedingly small numbers of microbes across the intestinal wall. Here, or in the local mesenteric lymph nodes (see Figure 10), they are dealt with by macrophages.

Lactobacilli are members of the normal intestinal flora, and more than a hundred years ago it was suggested they might be good for you. The great Elie Metchnikov (see pages 33–34) regarded the normal intestinal flora as 'toxic' and suggested replacing it with lactobacilli. He can be looked on as the founding father of the yoghurt industry. The jury is still out on the general health giving properties of lactobacilli, but they do alter the balance of microbes in the intestine. If children with diarrhoea are fed millions of lactobacilli every day the diarrhoea is less severe and they usually get better quicker. It is not clear how this works because the lactobacilli don't colonize the intestine, which is why they have to be given repeatedly, but the effect seems a genuine one.

Box 19 Reports from the rear

This is an opportunity to mention *flatus*. We all release 200–300 millilitres (half a pint) of gas each day from the mouth and anus. More than half of it is the nitrogen that was present in the air we have swallowed. We owe the rest to intestinal bacteria, which form hydrogen (H) and carbon dioxide (CO_2) gases and convert them to the gas methane (CH_4). The bacteria form larger amounts of gas in people that can't digest lactose (the sugar in milk), or when people eat beans. Overindulgence in beans can increase gas production ten-fold, although taking a pill (a 'beano' in the USA) containing raffinose helps digest the beans and prevents the build-up of gas. Otherwise, excessive wind-producing powers are due to the swallowing of air. The odour of flatus (as passed by posterior trumpeting) is another gift from intestinal bacteria and is caused by volatile substances such as hydrogen sulphide.

In the late 19th century Jean Pujol, a baker from Marseilles, France, gave flatus-based performances on the stage. He was known as 'Le Petomaine'. To packed houses he farted his way to fame, giving impressions of a trombone, a double bass, or of calico being torn, playing tunes on a tin flute and, with the aid of rubber tubing, smoking cigarettes. He could blow out a candle at 12 inches, and it was all based on his amazing capacity to draw in air through his anus and discharge it with superb control.

You might think that daily rubbing of millions of faecal bacteria into the skin round the anus with toilet paper would tend to cause infection. But it hardly ever does. Little is known about it because microbiologists have been reluctant to enter this interesting research area. Secretions from the prominent glands just inside the anus ooze over these regions and could have an antiseptic action. Alternatively the secretions may give mechanical protection merely by keeping the bacteria at a distance, like the mucus that tends to keep microbes away from the naked cells that line the intestine. The glands are surrounded by lymphocytes, and microbiologists might benefit from sailing these uncharted perianal seas.

Microbes in the skin

The skin is host to bacteria such as *Staphylococcus epidermidis* and the acne bacillus (see Glossary and pages 3–4, Chapter 1). Under a microscope they look like little heaps of rubble on a lunar landscape. They stick to skin scales and spread down from the surface as they divide, entering the mouths of hair follicles and glands. They are reduced in number, but never eliminated, by washing and scrubbing; within an hour or two they recolonize the surface as shown in Figure 17. In other words you can clean your hands and

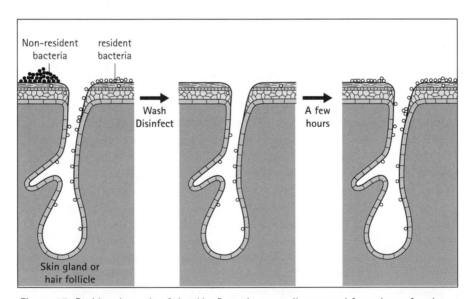

Figure 17 Resident bacteria of the skin. Bacteria are easily removed from the surface by washing or by antiseptics, but the residents deep down in skin glands and hair follicles are still there, and creep up to recolonize the surface within an hour or two.

remove harmful microbes, which is an excellent thing to do, the foundation for good hygiene and the prevention of infection. But you can't sterilize them (see Glossary) and get rid of the normal residents.

Most of the skin residents withstand drying and exposure to the salt from sweat glands, but larger numbers are found in moist areas like the armpit, groin and perineum. Feeding on substances that trickle out from sweat and on the oily material from sebaceous glands, they release odoriferous amines, which give us our characteristic body smell (see Box 20). The secretions have their own smell but the bacteria add that final bouquet. This is why many deodorants contain substances to stop bacterial growth. Odoriferous substances are formed by many bacteria and in the old days the bacteriologist always smelt his cultures as an aid to identifying them. Smell is superbly well-developed in dogs, and even in monkeys and apes it plays an important part in social and sexual life. At an early stage in human evolution, therefore, a personal body smell might have been looked upon as a benefit. Unexpectedly, there is a connection between smell and immune responses (see Box 20).

The smell of feet encased in socks is characteristic, and in many European

---

Box 20 Body odour examined

As a surprising twist to the story of smell, there is an association with the important MHC molecules described in Chapter 3 and Glossary. Many animals instinctively choose as a mate an unrelated individual. Humans tend to do the same thing, and observations of young people in kibbutzim in Israel showed that they usually chose marriage partners from other kibbutzim rather than from the lifelong companions in their own kibbutz. This makes biological sense because it mixes up genes and avoids inbreeding. In mice the actual preference seems to be for an individual carrying different MHC genes. This, too, makes sense, because by acquiring different MHC genes you also acquire the capacity to handle a wider variety of microbial antigens (see page 129, Part 3) and are less likely to be wiped out by a new pestilence.

So how do mice know about the MHC equipment of potential mates? It turns out that in mice the genes for MHC are closely associated with those for body odour, and an MHC-based choice can thus be achieved by smell! How much of this holds true for humans with our somewhat atrophied sense of smell is not clear.

languages is referred to as 'cheese-like'. Between the toes lives a certain bacterium responsible for the smell. A similar bacterium is added to cheeses like brie to enhance the flavour.

One interesting site for skin microbes is the area under the foreskin, the chosen haunt of another very specialized harmless resident, a bacterium related to tuberculosis bacteria. This moist backwater is easily contaminated by sexually transmitted microbes, giving them more opportunity to establish themselves, which is probably why uncircumcized men are more readily infected with HIV, syphilis and gonorrhoea.

The shedding of skin scales, most of them carrying resident bacteria, has been referred to on pages 97 and 140. Only small numbers are shed when we are motionless, but even slight activity increases the number ten-fold and vigorous activity a hundred-fold. Undressing is especially dangerous, with 1500–2000 bacteria per cubic foot discharged into the air.

The type of staphylococci that cause pimples, boils and styes are often normal residents, and likely to be present on the fingers, the 'nose-picking' zone in the nostrils and on the perineum, presumably carried to these areas by promiscuous digital probing (see Box 21).

Residents sometimes take liberties

The normal residents have established a balance with host defences. Any weakening of the latter allows residents to do things they would never normally be allowed to do. Many of the infections that plague hospitals are caused by resident bacteria that have taken the opportunities offered by defects in host defences. These are called *opportunist* infections. For example, we saw in Chapter 4 how a catheter in a vein or in the urethra allows the local skin or urogenital residents to enter the blood circulation or the bladder. And we also saw in Chapter 4 how defects in immune responses (steroids, AIDS) or in other defences (diabetes, cystic fibrosis) give further opportunities to residents.

All the residents are tolerated, somehow avoiding the immune attack that would expel less experienced microbes, and while they take liberties when our defences are crippled, they are of some use to us. By taking up the available space and by secreting substances that inhibit other microbes, they tend to keep out many of the potentially harmful ones. *E. coli* from the intestine cannot establish themselves in the mouth because of competition from the local inhabitants. Again, people given antibiotics such as tetracycline that act against the normal bacterial flora may suffer from overgrowth of the resident mould *Candida*, causing thrush in the mouth or vagina. *Candida*'s unbalanced growth is normally prevented by the other members of the flora.

> **Box 21   Pus and boils in the 1940s**
>
> In the days before antibiotics staphylococcal pus (see page 37, Chapter 2) was a regular sight. The matron at my boarding school in 1940 held a regular boil clinic, where boils, especially in the neck, were cleaned, squeezed, dressed, poulticed. Certain boys were regulars in the queue. Perhaps they were by nature susceptible to staphylococci, but those shirt collars must have been teeming with bacteria (we only changed shirts once a week) rubbed all day into adolescent necks.
>
> Larger collections of pus form abscesses. Once these have formed there is nothing for it but to cut open the abscess (lance it) and allow the pus to escape. In the old days half a pint of staphylococcal pus was often obtained from an abscess in the breast or on the backside (ischio-rectal abscess).
>
> Staphylococci have lived on humans since time began, causing pussy spots, boils, carbuncles, abscesses and sometimes the 'toxic' diseases described on page 165, Chapter 8. The unpleasant strains are called *Staphylococcus aureus* because their colonies growing on gelatin plates in the lab have a golden colour (Latin, *aureus* = golden). We can clear them out from our noses with mupirocin or chlorhexidine creams and we can kill them with antibiotics, but we still don't know exactly what molecules make them start behaving as enemies rather than harmless residents. It has been said that the golden hordes of Gengis Khan's (1162–1227) Mongolian warriors, who sacked and destroyed towns, putting all inhabitants to death, and whose conquests stretched from China to Europe, were less devastating, less invasive, than the golden hordes of *S. aureus*.

Troublesome poisons from intestinal residents?

How is it that in that great fermentation chamber, the bowel, bacteria flourish on such a prodigious scale without being expelled? This is an interesting question, so far unanswered by the immunologists. Furthermore, the bacteria are in direct contact with living cells and surely they release unpleasant substances for us to absorb into the body.

At one time it was fashionable to believe that toxins absorbed from the bowel were responsible for various diseases. The great Elie Metchnikov (see pages 33–34) was an enthusiast and in 1901 suggested removal of 'nearly the whole of the large intestine' in these diseases. Constipation was a dreaded condition, needing relief by a veritable armoury of laxative treatments. From the mere sight and smell of bowel contents it seemed obvious that here was a formidable source of disease-producing materials. In the 1920s a famous London surgeon, adopting Metchnikov's view, began to remove whole sections of the intestine as a treatment for vaguely defined illnesses characterized by headaches, backaches, tiredness, insomnia, depression, and so on. Even now, ritual washing out (irrigation) of the large bowel has its devotees. Diets with substantial amounts of fibre are popular, so that the gut contents move along less sluggishly, but in any case we are less worried about our bowel movements than were our grandfathers. Within reason, there is nothing inherently wrong with constipation! Think of the breastfed infant, who seems content with a bowel movement about once a week.

Undesirable residents

One or two microbes are present in so many normal people that they can perhaps be regarded as normal residents, yet they regularly cause disease. First there are the viruses such as those causing cold sores and chickenpox, described on pages 180–187, which are present in a latent form in most of us. They reside in nerve ganglia, ready to emerge and give us cold sores or shingles. Other less well-known viruses come into the same category and you, dear reader, have at the moment at least six different viruses tucked away in safe corners of your body, behaving themselves today but ready to cause mischief if given the opportunity. Second there is *Streptococcus mutans*, a regular resident but an indispensable microbial factor in tooth decay (caries, see below). Third, living in the stomach of more than half of us, is *Helicobacter pylori*, which causes peptic ulcers and whose adaptation to an acid environment is described on page 101.

A germ-free life?

What happens if there are no resident microbes on the skin, or in the mouth and intestines? In the laboratory we can produce animals (mice, pigs, cats, horses) that are totally sterile, devoid of the normal flora. To do this the young are removed from the mother by caesarean section, and immediately placed in a germ-free environment, supplied with sterile food, water and air. It is a technically demanding, expensive business, needing constant surveillance. Generally the germ-free animals live longer, and not unexpectedly their immune system is less well-developed, less well-exercised, because of the absence of microbes. They do not have to maintain that constant immune and inflammatory activity against intestinal microbes, and the gut wall is therefore quite thin.

From germ-free animals we have learnt a lot about infection and immunity. But the germ-free life is an impossibly artificial, expensive condition, technically demanding and psychologically crippling for an intelligent animal. We have to accept that colonization by the normal flora is our unavoidable fate. A more worthy aim would be to eliminate all the regularly harmful microbes. In developed countries we have already made some progress along this path and one day, with the help of vaccines, and as the other fruits of science are devoted to human wellbeing, it may be achieved.

HOW DISEASES ARE NAMED

When an infecting microbe makes us ill, we name the condition according to the organ that is affected, and the suffix '-itis' means that the organ is inflamed. Thus hepatitis for the liver, bronchitis for the bronchi, cystitis for the bladder, encephalitis for the brain, gastroenteritis for the stomach and intestines, and so on. The name of the disease generally tells us nothing about the actual cause. Hepatitis, for instance, can be due to at least six quite different viruses (hepatitis viruses A–F), meningitis to numerous viruses and bacteria and pneumonitis or pneumonia to a veritable army of microbes (viruses, bacteria, protozoa, fungi). Although some microbes, such as the hepatitis and influenza viruses, focus on one organ, others are less fussy. Herpes simplex virus (cold sores) invades skin, mucosal surfaces and the nervous system, and syphilis bacteria cause disease in so many different parts of the body that the great physician William Osler remarked that 'He who knows syphilis knows medicine.'

Not unexpectedly, damage to some organs has more impact on the host than damage to others. If a muscle in the shoulder is out of action for a week (myositis) it is not too serious, but our very existence depends on regular contractions of another great muscle, the heart, and here a small amount of damage (myocarditis) may be life-threatening. A slight amount of inflammation and swelling in the liver can be tolerated (indeed the liver has such reserves of function that you can remove half of it without ill effect) whereas the same amount of swelling in the brain, enclosed in a rigid box (the skull), is disastrous. This is why meningitis and encephalitis are such serious diseases, calling for emergency treatment.

It hardly needs to be said that the personal as well as the bodily impact of damage depends on where it occurs. When an unpleasant-looking discharge issues from the nose it can (according to present rules of conduct) be blown out into a handkerchief in public, whereas the emission of similar material from the urethra (gonorrhoea or chlamydial urethritis) is not likely to be heralded in this way. The latter type of discharge is also more uncomfortable, yet in essence it is no more than a cold in the urethra.

SIGNS AND SYMPTOMS

I keep on referring to the age-old conflict between microbial invaders and host defences. It takes two to make a disease, as it does to make a quarrel. Often the outcome of the conflict is an unnoticed episode of infection with no significant damage with development of immunity. A large proportion of all infections are in this category. Most virus infections are silent, private, battles between the invader and the immune system, unnoticed by the person in whose body they are taking place.

Alternatively the outcome can be a disease. But there is a spectrum. Even conditions that have a bad-sounding name such as poliomyelitis or Japanese encephalitis are asymptomatic in most people, infection being detected only by the appearance in the blood of antibodies. Those with paralysis (polio) or encephalitis (Japanese encephalitis) represent the tip of the iceberg. Box 22 summarizes the whole of infectious disease as the result of the microbe–host conflict.

Admittedly there are one or two microbes that cause a characteristic and serious disease in virtually every infected individual, for example rabies, bubonic plague, or HIV. Even measles causes a standard type of illness in all children, although it varies greatly in severity. On the other hand mumps, such an easily diagnosed disease that we have no trouble recognizing Hippocrates' description of it 2500 years ago, is often asymptomatic. The child (and the mother) then quite rightly maintains that he has never had mumps, meaning the disease, but he was nevertheless infected with the virus and has developed immunity. To put the possibilities in an irreverent nutshell:

> *'You have two choices – one of getting the germ and one of not. And if you get the germ you have two choices – one of getting the disease and one of not. And if you get the disease you have two choices – one of dying and one of not. And if you die you still have two choices!'*
>
> (Anon)

Box 22 Seeing both points of view in an infectious disease

THE CONFLICT

	The host's point of view – defend	The microbe's point of view – invade
Outer defences	Physical barriers	Stick to body surfaces, enter via bite or wound
	Surface cleaning	Interfere with cleaning
Early defences	Inflammation	Avoid starting it
	Phagocytes	Don't get taken up and killed, or kill the phagocyte
	Interferon, etc.	Stop it being formed or resist it
Immune defences	Antibody	Evade antibodies, stop them acting
	Cell-mediated immunity	Interfere with development or action of immune responses

RESULT OF THE CONFLICT

	Verdict for host		Verdict for microbe
Early defences victorious	Success	No invasion no disease	Failure
Immune defences victorious after microbe has done what it wants	Success	Invasion and shedding of microbe but no disease	Success
Host victory after successful invader has caused disease	Success	Invasion, disease, microbial shedding, but recovery	Success
Defences inadequate or immune response does too much damage	Failure	Invasion, disease, death +/- microbial shedding	Success*

* Success if there is shedding, but severe disease or death would make this a less successful outcome if it depleted the host species.

For all infectious diseases the exact clinical picture depends on the particular strain of the microbe, and this is important for many infections, but not, as it happens, for measles or mumps. It also depends on age, sex, nutrition and the other factors that influence host defences (see Part 2).

THE BIG KILLERS

To put things in perspective I am going to start with the worst infections, the biggest killers of human beings. Remember that an infection can be highly lethal, yet not all that common, so that the total impact on humanity is quite small. There are many dramatic infections in this category, such as Ebola fever and rabies. Ebola virus has been the exciting subject of a book and a Dustin Hoffman movie called *Outbreak*. It kills most people that get it, but it is restricted to certain parts of Africa and the total number of deaths so far is less than a thousand.

Let us consider *rabies*. It is one of the oldest and most feared of human diseases, and was known more than 4000 years ago. The case of Rajam in India was described on pages 7–8, Chapter 1. Rabies virus naturally infects foxes, jackals, dogs, wolves, cats, skunks, raccoons and (in Central and South America) vampire bats. Its behaviour in these animals is admirably suited to its life-style.

The virus appears in the saliva and is transferred to other individuals during biting, or by licking small wounds. It then enters nerve endings in muscle and skin and travels slowly up the nerves, eventually reaching the spinal cord and brain. Here it does two important things. First, it spreads down the appropriate nerves to reach the salivary glands, where it multiplies and is discharged in large amounts into saliva. Second, it invades that part of the brain (the limbic system) that controls behaviour and, without actually destroying nerve cells, causes subtle alterations. The infected animal becomes more aggressive, more likely to bite another individual. In Russia, for instance, rabid wolves become agitated, desert their packs, and run up to 80 km a day, attacking livestock and people. But the rabid animal nearly always dies. The invasion of the limbic system seems to be nothing less than a fiendish survival strategy on the part of the virus, aimed at ensuring its own wide transmission and survival.

In humans, however, rabies virus reaches a *dead end*, as it generally does in other non-biting animals such as cattle, horses and sheep. After a person has been bitten by a rabid animal the infection can be halted in its tracks by giving rabies antibody or vaccine during the virus' lengthy journey up the nerves to the spinal cord and brain. But once the actual disease develops it is fatal, and the symptoms are often terrifying. In about half of human cases there is spasm of the throat and choking when attempting to drink, and this can be brought on by the mere sight of water – hence the name *hydrophobia*. Altogether there are about 75,000 cases of human rabies each year, mostly caused by dogs. It occurs throughout the world, with the exception of countries like Australia, New Zealand, Japan, UK, Finland, Sweden and Norway, where rigorous public health measures are enforced. Rabies is a terrible disease but numerically unimportant compared with the top killers now to be mentioned.

Today's top ten

Here we will be talking about numbers, and to put things in perspective we need to bear in mind the size of the world's population. In October 1999 it reached six billion (6,000,000,000) and now each week there is a surplus of births over deaths of nearly two million. In developing countries it has been calculated that up to one in four births is unwanted and 35 million abortions are performed yearly. Humans, at the level of governments, show a disinclination to attend to numbers when by their sheer numbers human beings have come to be a colossal global burden. Experts discuss the 'overloading of the biosphere', arguing as to whether supplies of water, food or power will run out first.

In the past 50 years more people have died from malaria, tuberulosis and AIDS than from all the wars combined. Infectious and parasitic diseases are the biggest killers of human beings, by sheer numbers. Nearly ten million people died in 1998, not from the exotic infections mentioned in Part 5, but from a few old-fashioned ones. The great majority of the deaths are in developing or the 'least developed' countries, where poor hygiene, malnutrition, lack of antibiotics and good medical services, make the infections more lethal. *All these things are due to poverty.* The world's economy continues to grow, yet around 1.3 billion people still live in total, grinding poverty on less than US$1 per day. And it is mostly children that die. Let us consider the top four killers, worldwide, not forgetting that death is not the only measure of human suffering (Box 23).

Respiratory (lung) infections are the worst culprits, accounting for the death of 3.5 million in 1998, most of them children under the age of five. The WHO is doing wonders with vaccines against whooping cough, diphtheria, measles, etc., but it is only in wealthy, developed countries that these diseases have been properly controlled.

AIDS (HIV). At the beginning of 1998, worldwide, about 30 million people

---

Box 23 The global burden of suffering

Death awaits us all, and is the only certain thing about life. Also, death is easy to count. But what about the great load of human suffering caused by years of disease or disability? Can we measure this? Recently scientists have been calculating something called DALY (Disability Adjusted Life Years). This is made up not only of the total years of life lost because of early death, but also the years spent suffering from diseases and disabilities, in other words Disability Adjusted Lost Years. The calculation is difficult but the results interesting.

We find that certain conditions such as major depression rank high on the DALY scale, whereas other diseases among the top causes of death rank lower when charted on the DALY scale.

Death and suffering in the world; 1998 figures (WHO Annual Report 1999)*

Deaths (millions)		DALY (millions of years lost)	
Heart disease	7.4	Pneumonia, etc.	82.3
Stroke	5.1	Perinatal conditions	80.6
Pneumonia, etc.	3.5	Diarrhoea	73.1
AIDS (HIV)	2.3	AIDS (HIV)	70.9
Chronic lung disease	2.3	Depression	58.2
Diarrhoea	2.2	Heart disease	51.9
Birth-related	2.2	Stroke	41.6
Tuberculosis	1.5	Malaria	39.3
Cancer of lung **	1.2	Traffic accidents	38.8
Traffic accidents***	1.2	Measles	30.2

* Total deaths from infectious and parasitic diseases in 1998 were 9.8 million, the DALY score being 295.7 million.

** Total cancer deaths were 7.2 million.

*** These are road traffic deaths. Total deaths by accident were 5.8 million, scoring 156.2 million years by DALY. Total 'intentional' deaths, by suicide, homicide, war, were 2.3 million, scoring 65.5 million years by DALY.

---

were infected with HIV, and 2.2 million died of AIDS in that year. More than 14 million have died of it since the epidemic began. Yet to put it in perspective, during the great 1918 influenza pandemic (see page 120) at least

20 million were killed in a mere two years, more than died during WW1 itself. Three-quarters of the HIV infections have been from unprotected sexual intercourse, and three-quarters of these were heterosexual. Infants and children are infected in the womb or in early infancy.

For its total impact one has to remember that although AIDS kills mainly young adults, it leaves orphans behind, and it makes people much more susceptible to tuberculosis, so that in Africa about one in three AIDS patients die of tuberculosis. AIDS deaths are about twice those due to motor cars (1.1 million), and this can be compared with the 1.7 million who committed suicide or were murdered.

HIV has not yet finished with the human race, and is taking its toll in India, Russia and China, as well as in sub-Saharan Africa, where more that one in ten people are infected. Note that AIDS, in contrast to respiratory and diarrhoeal infections, kills mainly adults.

Diarrhoeal infections. These come close behind AIDS. In 1988 2.2 million children died with diarrhoea, which works out at nearly 7000 deaths a day. There are parts of Africa, Asia and Latin America where the average 2–3-year-old child has diarrhoea for a total of 2–3 months a year. Some die, and others suffer stunted growth. The diarrhoea is due to a great variety of microbes and other parasites (see the story of Ricardo on pages 6–7), and the children show repeated troughs in their growth curves as they encounter the different intestinal microbes, many of which (such as amoebic dysentery and roundworms, see Glossary) have been banished from developed countries. Children with severe diarrhoea die easily because of the water and salt lost from their small bodies. When mothers give them drinks containing salt and sugar the death rate is greatly reduced. This a low-tech treatment with a big payoff.

The enormous amount of diarrhoea is mostly due to unclean water supplies and inadequate sewage disposal. About half the world's population cannot safely dispose of their bodily waste – their sewage disposal is inadequate. Such people live in mediaeval squalor and intestinal infections spread easily through these communities. And yet $6 million spent over ten years could solve the problem, a mere 1% of the global military budget!

In earlier centuries diarrhoea was a common cause of death in European children, especially during summer time. Records show that in London between 1667 and 1720, 328,234 infants died from summer diarrhoea, often described as 'griping of the guts'. An epitaph in a churchyard in Cheltenham, England, refers to an infant dying at the age of three weeks:

> *'It is so soon that I am done for,*
> *I wonder what I was begun for'*

Tuberculosis is now fourth in the list, accounting for 1.5 million deaths in 1998. We have the vaccine and the drugs that could largely overcome tuberculosis; the problem is that many poor countries cannot afford them and lack the means for delivering them to people. How do you ensure that a Somali nomad in Africa continues taking the medicine for the necessary six months? He will stop as soon as he feels better, and the tuberculosis bacteria, those great hangers-on, will re-emerge at a later date and make him ill again and able to infect others.

Increasing numbers of those with tuberculosis also have AIDS, especially in Africa. There is a sinister synergy between AIDS and tuberculosis, and together they form a lethal combination.

For comparison it can be noted that in 1998 tobacco was responsible for four million deaths worldwide, more than any of the top four infectious and parasitic killers.

The next commonest killers, after the top four, are:

Millions dead in 1998 (WHO figures)

Malaria	1.1	Ninety per cent of the deaths are in Africa, nearly all in children under the age of five. There is now no reliable preventative drug and you just have to avoid mosquito bites.
Measles	0.9	Still great killers of children in
Whooping cough	0.35	developing countries, though preventable by the vaccines.
Tetanus of the newborn	0.4	Due to bacteria from the soil entering the cut surface of the umbilical cord.
Syphilis	0.16	
Meningitis	0.14	
Sleeping sickness	0.15	Spread by tsetse flies in Africa (see pages 109–111).
Hepatitis	0.009	But note that hepatitis B causes liver cancer, which killed 0.6 million.

Note also that I have not included Lassa fever, Ebola fever, schistosomiasis, cholera, typhus, rabies, poliomyelitis and a host of other well-known and often lethal infections in my list of big killers. This is because numerically they are less important than the ones I have mentioned. They can be dramatic and newsworthy, but are not major causes of death, worldwide.

BIG KILLERS FROM LONG AGO

One or two epidemics have found a place in recorded history, generally because of their effect on armies and military activities. Total numbers killed may seem small by today's standards but the impact was great. The Plague of Athens, for instance, in 430–429 BC, killed off about a quarter of the Athenian land army. It came from Ethiopia, via Egypt, and disappeared as mysteriously as it came. Athenian society never completely recovered. Again, when in 701 BC a fatal and presumably infectious disease suddenly attacked the Assyrians, 185,000 of them are said to have died and Sennaccherib, their king, had to withdraw his army from Judah without conquering Jerusalem. The episode is immortalized in Lord Byron's poem 'The Destruction of Sennaccherib'.

Unfortunately it is impossible to identify most of these infections from historical accounts. Was it influenza, measles, typhus, dysentery? Nothing short of a time machine is likely to help us. We are perhaps on firmer ground with the epidemic described by a Chinese doctor Ko Hung (281–361 AD), who wrote of '...epidemic sores that attack head, face, or trunk...with the appearance of hot boils containing white matter...those who recover are disfigured by purplish scars...'. Because this epidemic was encountered by Chinese armies when they attacked the barbarians at Nan-Yung it was called 'Barbarian Pox', and it sounds like smallpox (see page 155), which came to China from the northwest sometime between 37 and 653 AD.

The English Sweating Sickness of the 15th to 16th century is described on page 16. The *plague* has long been an accepted big killer (see Box 24).

Goodbye to smallpox

From the beginning of recorded history, smallpox has been a killer. Kings died of it, and when 15th to 18th century explorers and colonists introduced it into Africa, the Americas and Australia, the impact was comparable to that of guns and the Bible. In the Aztec and Inca kingdoms an estimated 3.5 million died within a few years. The fact that the Spanish

---

Box 24 The plague in a nutshell

For thousands of years the plague bacteria (*Yersinia pestis*) have existed in rodents in the Far East, which are their chosen hosts, occasionally spreading to humans to cause epidemics. In January 1348, three galleys, laden with spices from the East, brought the plague to the port of Genoa, Italy. The disease then spread to the rest of Europe and arrived in London in December 1348. Conditions here were ideal, with at least one family of black rats per household and three fleas to a rat. Black rats are ideal for spreading the plague. The infection kills this type of rat and as the corpse cools the fleas desert it to find fresh food (blood) and lodging on human bodies.

Because it was winter the infection soon began to spread directly from person to person by respiratory (droplet) infection, with a speed and violence that was terrifying. People died in their thousands, rich and poor alike. To the mediaeval mind it seemed that a miasma, a poison, was responsible, and infected houses were labelled and boarded up, together with the inhabitants. The population of England at this time was about four million, and over a period of two and a half years about a third of them (more than a million) died.

The bacteria, introduced into the body by the bite of the rat flea, multiply and invade the local lymph nodes in the armpit or groin to give bubonic plague (Greek, *bubo* = groin). The nodes are soon destroyed and turn into bags of pus. Meanwhile the bacteria have spread through the rest of the body, releasing their toxins and soon killing the patient. When plague bacteria invade the lungs (pneumonic plague) the infection can be spread by droplets and explosive, devastating outbreaks are possible. The disease, which became known as The Black Death, was attributed to earthquakes, to the movements of the planets, to a Jewish or Arab plot (350 massacres of Jews took place during the epidemic years in Europe), and most commonly to God's punishment for human wickedness.

Another epidemic in 1665, the year before the Great Fire of London, was graphically described by Daniel Defoe (who was only five years old at the time) in his *Journal of a Plague Year in London*.

> 'They had dug several pits in another ground, when
> the distemper began to spread in our parish, and
> especially when the dead carts began to go about,...
> Into these pits they had put perhaps fifty or sixty
> bodies each; then they made larger holes, wherein

> Box 24 The plague in a nutshell (continued)
>
> > *they buried all that the cart brought in a week,*
> > *which...came to from 200 to 400 a week; and they*
> > *could not well dig them larger, because of the*
> > *order of the magistrates confining them to leave*
> > *no bodies within six feet of the surface.'*
>
> The last plague epidemic arose in China and reached Hong Kong in 1894, where Yersin (and independently Kitasato) identified and described the causative bacterium. Infected rodents are still present in many parts of the world, including western USA, but the disease is uncommon, with only 2000 cases worldwide in 1993. It can be cured or prevented by antibiotics, yet when it spreads by droplets it can still bring out that mediaeval fear of contagion that lies in all of us, as was apparent in the 1994 outbreak in Surat, India. People wore masks, fled the cities, and airports throughout the world were alerted.

conquistadores were resistant, having already encountered the disease in Spain and developed immunity, made them seem even more invincible.

The disease was due to a large virus, wonderfully equipped with devices for overcoming immune defences. Infection generally took place when droplets were inhaled during face-to-face contact, and the virus then carried out a step by step invasion of the body, rather like measles (see Figure 19). Smallpox was a regular feature of life in the towns and cities of Europe 200 years ago. For children it was like the measles, a hurdle to be got over, and it caused about a third of all childhood deaths. Smallpox scars were common, one in three Londoners were scarred, while milkmaids enjoyed a reputation for unblemished complexions. People learnt that you could protect against smallpox by scratching into skin the material from the blisters (pocks) of sufferers, and Lady Wortley Montague, wife of the British Ambassador to Turkey, brought this method back with her to England, where it was widely used. In 1722 two Royal princesses were protected in this way, after preliminary tests on six condemned criminals from Newgate Prison (see pages 43–44, Chapter 3).

Seventy-five years later a country doctor of enquiring mind, Edward Jenner, who lived in Berkeley, Gloucester, England, discovered the modern vaccine for smallpox. On May 14, 1796, he took material from a cowpox blister on the hand of a dairymaid, Sarah Nelmes (who had caught it from a cow called Blossom), and rubbed it into scratches made on the arm of 8-year-old James Phipps. James suffered a very mild indisposition, and six weeks later Jenner inoculated him with virulent smallpox material. The boy remained well. It was a risky thing to do, but the boy had been protected. It was not until 87 years later that the next vaccine, against rabies, was developed by Louis Pasteur.

Jenner was not so rushed as today's GPs, and found time to be a keen biologist as well as a physician. He studied temperature changes in hibernating animals, the breeding of toads and eels, and was first to describe the way the cuckoo nestling ejects the eggs and young of the foster parents from the nest.

Jenner's method was called vaccination (Latin, *vacca* = cow), and by the first half of the 20th century smallpox had been almost eradicated from Europe and North America. But the disease continued in Asia and Africa and as late as 1974 there were nearly a quarter of a million cases.

In 1969 the WHO began a campaign to wipe out smallpox, using Jenner's vaccine. There were daunting difficulties, such as cultural barriers, warfare and transport to remote areas. How do you get to villages in the highlands of Ethiopia that are more than 20 miles from the nearest tracks negotiable by Land Rover? However, the campaign was eventually successful and the last case of smallpox was in October 1977 in a small town in Somalia, Africa. Smallpox has now gone forever, it is an extinct species.

The total cost of the campaign, arguably the greatest achievement of medical science in the 20th century, was US $150 million. For it to be successfully eradicated the disease had to be:

- An exclusively human one. If it infected animals or insects it could come back again.

- One that did not stay around in the body; if it did, it would mean there could be healthy carriers.

- There had to be a good and cheap vaccine. Jenner's vaccine fitted the bill, although, by the way, it would not even be licensed by today's strict standards.

- There had to be the resources and organization to carry it through on a global scale. For smallpox this was provided by the WHO and its devoted band of scientists, administrators, vaccinators and epidemiologists.

Chapter 8

HOW MICROBES CAUSE DISEASE

MOST MICROBES DON'T

As often as not, microbes do not cause disease. I have already described the members of the normal flora and they are generally well-behaved. Even with those microbes that do cause disease there is a whole spectrum of responses, and without overstating it one could say that in most people (meaning more than half of them) most infections are symptomless. The occasional person who is ill represents the tip of the iceberg and the majority undergo an inapparent infection. Epstein–Barr (EB) virus in small children (see page 175) is a good example.

Warts, our ancient companions, are almost harmless
I was passing through Kuala Lumpur in 1982 and visited the big mosque, taking off my shoes and socks, as is customary, before entering and walking about on the damp stone floors. Three months after returning home, two warts (verrucas) appeared on the soles of my feet. I let them be because they were not uncomfortable, and eventually, after 5–6 months, they disappeared.

Warts are exceedingly ancient human parasites, our constant companions for millions of years. Their success is reflected in the fact that there are more than 60 different types of human wart virus. Only a small number of these are really common; the rest are rarely seen. Indeed two of them have been found exclusively in American Indians and in Inuits.

It would be stretching a point to say that warts cause diseases, apart from the genital wart connection with cancer (see page 179), which is their main claim to fame. Warts are humble. As a group, however, they are admirable parasites, more securely attached to our surfaces than limpets to rocks, yet causing next to no trouble. To be so successful they have needed a strategy, and this is outlined in Box 25.

For a wart virus, the skin is a vast empire in which the different territories and climates are almost as varied as those on the earth itself. Certain types of wart virus go for the fingers and knuckles, spreading to the lips particularly in nail-biters and thumb-suckers. Others have adapted to life on the soles of the feet, causing the plantar warts described above, and because a mature wart is a lump protruding from the skin the weight of the body presses the plantar wart deep into the skin and sometimes makes it uncomfortable to walk. The rough non-slip edges of swimming pools are good spreaders of plantar warts.

Nine or ten different types of wart virus have jumped onto the STD (sexually transmitted disease) bandwagon, and are spread by mucosal contacts.

Box 25 How warts get round immune defences

We become infected by way of unnoticed abrasions on the skin or mucosa. These surfaces consist of several layers of cells, and the virus enters the deepest layer, the cells that are constantly dividing to compensate for those sloughed off from the surface as skin scales. The virus stays here, but only in the form of its DNA; no antigens or infectious material are formed until the cells begin to move up towards the surface. Fully fledged wart viruses appear, with perfect timing, when the cells have flattened, turned into dry scales of keratin, and are about to be shed from the body (see Figure 14). This means that down below, nearer to prowling T cells and antibodies, the virus sits snugly inside cells and cannot be identified.

It takes a long time for the first infected cell to give rise to a crop of descendant cells large enough to be seen as a wart, and therefore the average incubation period before it is visible is 3–4 months, and sometimes it can be as long as a year or more. In the end the CMI arm of the immune system catches up with the invader and the warts vanish, often all at the same time. The latest remedy is given the credit. The DNA of the virus, however, tends to stay in cells in the deepest layers of the skin. When immune defences are weakened, for instance during the immunosuppressive treatment given after a kidney transplant, the virus wakes up from its long sleep, and crops of warts may appear, which seem to come from nowhere.

In the cervix and vagina they cause only flat patches, but they cause proper warts on the vulva, penis, and the area round the anus. Here they are noticed rather than suffered from, although they occasionally burn or itch. Warts on the penis range from those that are so small as to be invisible to the naked eye, to cauliflower-like protuberances of an ornamental nature.

The treatment for warts is to remove them, either by applying a gently acting substance like podophyllin, or by freezing them with liquid nitrogen (minus 180°C!), or (in the cervix) by burning them out with a laser.

So far no one has discovered a good way of growing wart viruses in the laboratory, and scientifically, therefore, warts languished in the stone age until the flowering of molecular biology 30 years ago. Now their DNA can be studied and we have learnt a lot about them. Also about unexpected things. DNA studies on warts from many different countries have enabled scientists to say that human wart viruses evolved along five distinct lines. The root of origin was in Africa, and there are now two African, plus European, Japanese/Chinese, and Asian lineages, whose courses parallel the history and migration of human beings over the past few million years. This is viral archaeology and it shows that warts are indeed ancient human companions!

Homage to lymphocytic choriomeningitis virus
We have to go to mice for a near perfect example of a benign invader, one so well-behaved that it establishes itself permanently in all cells and organs of the host without doing any damage. This is lymphocytic choriomeningitis (LCM) virus, and it has been exceptionally well-studied by scientists. When you examine infected cells under the electron microscope you can see the virus being released, but otherwise these cells look perfectly normal. Mice are infected right from the start of their embryonic life, because the virus is already present in the ovary and the eggs of the mother. It therefore gets into all the embryo cells and organs, including the thymus gland during its development. Having the virus multiply in the developing thymus means (see pages 50–51, Chapter 4) that virus materials (antigens) are regarded as 'self' rather than foreign and the T cells that might have reacted with them are eliminated. There is therefore no immune response to the infection. LCM virus continues to grow in the mouse throughout its life, causing no damage but constantly excreted in saliva, urine and faeces.

The picture of a 'tolerant' immune system and no damage to cells tells us that under these circumstances LCM is an ancient infection of mice, well-adapted to its host. However, if in the laboratory the virus is introduced into an adult mouse that has not been infected from birth, there is a vigorous immune response. Lymphocytes (T cells) pour into the sites of infection, and in the brain this leads to a fatal inflammation of the coverings (meninges) and the lining (choroid) of the brain. This is lymphocytic choriomeningitis (LCM). The T cells do their job and the virus is eliminated, but the accompanying inflammation, in this particular part of the body, is enough to kill the mouse. The disease is entirely due to the immune response because the virus infection itself does no damage, and if the immune response is prevented by giving an immunosuppressive drug, the infected mouse remains well.

Unfortunately LCM virus, so harmless in mice when they are infected under natural circumstances as embryos, can cause an unpleasant disease in humans. This used to happen when mice in an apartment block were infected, all mice carrying the virus and excreting it in their urine. Food was easily contaminated by the urine, and people became infected. The virus infects the same parts of the human brain as it does in the artificially infected adult mouse, and large numbers of lymphocytes are attracted, resulting in a LCM.

LCM virus is one of a group of at least a dozen very similar viruses, each causing a harmless infection in a certain species of rodent in a certain part of the world. If humans are exposed to the urine of these rodents and are infected, the disease can be serious. Examples include Lassa fever virus (in West Africa), and the viruses of Argentinian and Bolivian Haemorrhagic fevers (see Part 5).

THE MICROBE RELEASES A TOXIN

Many microbes, with the exception of the smallest ones (viruses), release substances into the body as they multiply. Some of these substances are formed as part of the microbe's strategy, because they interfere with host defences, as outlined in Part 3, and others are no more than mere by-products of microbial growth. However, a few of these substances, called toxins, have a dramatic damaging action on the host.

Three famous toxins

The diseases tetanus, diphtheria and cholera are caused by toxic molecules (toxins) formed by the infecting bacteria. If they didn't form the toxin these bacteria would be harmless.

Tetanus

The bacteria causing tetanus (*Clostridium tetani*) live in the intestines of domestic animals (and humans), and are excreted in faeces as spores. A spore is a highly resistant form of the microbe, not inactivated by boiling, or by disinfectants like phenol. Tetanus spores are therefore ubiquitous in soil, particularly in places where there are large animals such as horses. They cause trouble when introduced into the body's tissues, and because they grow best in the absence of oxygen (are anaerobic, see Glossary) they prefer damaged or dying tissues, where there is a shortage of oxygen.

The opportunity comes when soil containing the bacterial spores contaminates a wound, especially when it also contains a piece of foreign material like a fragment of soil or clothing. The wound may be small, such as a splinter or thorn in the finger, or it may be the umbilical stump of a newborn baby. Sometimes it is a larger wound, for instance the lining of the uterus after an abortion, or a major injury sustained on the battlefield or in a car crash.

The bacterial spores now come to life, start to grow in the damaged tissues, and release their toxin, which travels up local nerves to reach the spinal cord and brain. Here it acts on the nerve cells that control muscle contraction, causing uncontrollable convulsive movements. Spasm often begins, alarmingly, in eye muscles or jaw muscles (lockjaw), and eventually spreads to the muscles used in breathing. About half of all patients with tetanus die of exhaustion or pneumonia unless they are treated by injecting them with antibodies (antitoxin) to neutralize the toxin (see page 64).

In most parts of the world children are now given the excellent vaccine, which is injected into the arm and makes them produce their own antibodies to the toxin. Tetanus is therefore very uncommon. In developing countries, however, tens of thousands of newborn children each year still die of tetanus, because the umbilical stump gets contaminated by soil or by dirty instruments used to cut the umbilical cord.

Diphtheria

This is my second disease caused by a toxin. In this disease the bacterium (*Corynebacterium diphtheriae*) colonizes the nose, throat and windpipe (sometimes the skin), but without penetrating very deeply below the surface. An exceedingly powerful toxin is released, so powerful that a single molecule of it can kill a cell. The toxin is useful to the bacteria because it destroys local cells and helps the bacteria get established on the surface of the body. They can then multiply and spread to other people by means of droplets. By itself this local damage might not matter, but unfortunately it results in considerable inflammation and swelling, with formation of a membrane-like piece of dead tissue (Greek, *diphthera* = membrane). When this occurs in the windpipe it can interfere with breathing to such an extent that the patient chokes to death. Sixty years ago, before widespread use of the diphtheria vaccine, many infectious disease hospitals had an alarm bell for use when a child arrived in an ambulance, fighting for breath, dying of diphtheria. Emergency treatment was by cutting into the windpipe in the front of the neck, below the obstruction, and inserting a tube through which life-saving air could be breathed.

Unfortunately in this disease, there was often more to come. The same toxin, when it spread round the body, had harmful effects on nerves and on the heart. The child might now, especially if the bacteria had colonized the throat (a good place for absorbing the toxin), develop paralysis of the swallowing muscles or inflammation of the heart (myocarditis, see Box 26). As with tetanus, treatment of diphtheria was by giving antibody to the toxin (antitoxin) and it could be life-saving. The first time diphtheria antitoxin was used in England was by Sir Arthur Sherrington in 1894. He had in his stables one of the first horses to be used to produce the antibody and one evening heard that his seven-year-old nephew was very ill with diphtheria. He bled this horse by candlelight, and the next morning drove in a dog-cart to his brother-in-law's house and injected the serum into his nephew. The boy recovered and 'grew to be six feet tall'.

Box 26 A schoolboy gets diphtheria in the 1930s

I caught diphtheria in 1935, and was moved from boarding school to an isolation hospital, one where visitors were allowed no nearer than the ground outside the windows, communication being by waving and smiling. Lying in bed one day, feeling slightly better, I sat up, only to lose consciousness immediately and fall back onto the pillow. The diphtheria toxin had acted on the heart, making it unable to pump enough blood up to the brain when I was in a sitting position.

After recovering from the illness I was found still to be carrying the diphtheria bacteria in my throat. This meant isolation in the school sanatorium, undergoing regular throat swabs which were tested for the presence of the bacteria, followed by painting the throat with a disgusting disinfectant fluid. I had to stay in the school sanatorium for a whole term, and there was nothing to do except read comics and one or two books. This must have been my introduction to solitary reading.

Nowadays diphtheria, like tetanus, is totally preventable by giving the vaccine, and the child forms antibodies that will neutralize the toxin. Nothing more is needed for resistance to these diseases.

From the point of view of the microbe the actions of the diphtheria toxin on nerves and on heart seem to serve no useful function, and they therefore can be thought of as unfortunate accidents. The bacteria should be asked to apologize. Tetanus toxin, also, seems of no value to the microbe, and it is interesting that in each case the toxin is not produced by the actual bacteria, but by a virus (phage) that parasitizes the bacterium. In a way, the bacteria are innocent.

Cholera

This is the third disease due to a toxin (see Box 27). In this case the bacterium (*Vibrio cholerae*) is taken in with drink or food. It is a successful intestinal microbe, and attaches to cells lining the intestinal wall and begins to multiply. It now releases a toxin that interferes with the working of cells without damaging them. The affected cells allow water and salts to leak through from the body into the gut. At first the rest of the intestine can cope by reabsorbing these materials but as the bacteria multiply and more and more cells are involved, this becomes impossible. As a result the patient with cholera suffers a profuse watery diarrhoea, as much as a litre an hour. In the face of such a massive loss of fluid and salts the circulation collapses,

---

Box 27 The story of cholera

For hundreds of years this disease has rampaged across Asia and the Middle East, spread by faecally contaminated water. Early strains of bacteria were recovered by bacteriologists from the dead bodies of pilgrims returning from Mecca. When cholera came to the crowded, insanitary cities of Europe and America in the 1830s it had a devastating effect. In the 1831 outbreak in England 60,000 people died.

The cholera outbreaks in London, in retrospect, had some beneficial side-effects. The river Thames in those days was little more than a sewer, receiving the cities' faecal discharges in untreated form, with water intake pipes often a short distance downstream from the sewage exit. Perfect conditions for a faecal–oral type of microbe! It was a London whose squalor was described by Charles Dickens in *Oliver Twist*. No one understood where the disease came from, and during the outbreaks in the 1860s cannon

---

Box 27 The story of cholera (continued)

were discharged regularly to clear the air of the 'miasmas' that were thought to be responsible. Members of Parliament in the House of Commons overlooking the river were familiar with the disgusting odours from the river banks, especially at low tide, but they could hold a lavender-soaked handkerchief to the nose. However, faced with the mounting death rate from cholera they were more receptive to the pleas from Edwin Chadwick and other social reformers that something should be done about the appalling sanitary conditions in the city. Chadwick published his *Report on The Sanitary Condition of the Labouring Population of Great Britain* in 1842, and an Act for Promoting Public Health was passed in 1848. As a result the full genius of Victorian engineering was directed to the construction of efficient sewage and fresh water supply systems (see also page 235).

Another beneficial effect of the cholera outbreaks in London was that they gave the opportunity for a great step forward in our understanding of infectious disease. In 1854 Dr John Snow charted on a map the cholera cases in his London practice, and noticed that all of them used the same pump in Broad Street, Soho, for their water supply. He had the handle of the pump removed, and the outbreak was terminated. From this experiment he concluded that the disease came from water and decided that it was spread from person to person after multiplying in the sufferer. This was long before the actual bacterium causing cholera was isolated by Koch (1883). Snow was also a pioneer in anaesthesia. On April 7 1853 he records in his diary that at the birth of Prince Leopold to Queen Victoria, in her apartment: 'I commenced to give a little chloroform with each pain, by pouring about 15 minims (drops) by measure on a folded handkerchief.'

Cholera still causes dramatic outbreaks, mainly in developing countries, but it is responsible for only a tiny fraction of the world's total diarrhoea deaths. In 1995 the first person to be infected in Europe for more than ten years got the disease by drinking fresh coconut milk imported from Thailand. And of course even when someone has the disease, the infection can no longer spread in our hygienic towns and cities.

In 1856 another general practitioner, Dr William Budd, studied the typhoid cases in his village, North Tawton, near Bristol, and decided that typhoid fever was another disease spread by faecal contamination of drinking water. He was clear about the infectiousness of faeces and noted that '...the sewer is, so to speak, the direct continuation of the diseased intestine'. And in the USA a book dealer, Lemuel Shattuck, following in Chadwick's footsteps, transformed the state of sanitation in Massachusetts.

leading to death a mere 12–24 hours after being taken ill. This could be the disease referred to in the Bible: 'I am poured out like water and all my bones are out of joint; my heart is like wax; it is melted away in the midst of my bowels.' (Psalms 22;14.) The patient's life can be saved if the lost fluids and salts are replaced by injecting (transfusing) them into a vein.

Toxins in other diseases

Toxins are important in various other diseases, including food-poisoning, anthrax, botulism and scarlet fever (see Glossary). *Staphylococcus* is worth mentioning here because certain strains of the genus form toxins that give rise to three different diseases.

The scalded skin syndrome
This affects infants, who are not very ill, but it is an alarming condition because large areas of skin (the outer layers) flake off, leaving normal skin underneath. The staphylococcal toxin that causes the disease disrupts the cement that normally keeps the different layers of skin together.

Toxic shock syndrome
This is a rare complication of staphylococcal infection, anywhere in the body, which became well-known after it was shown to occur in women using vaginal tampons. The especially absorbent material in the tampons became contaminated with the bacteria, and as the toxin was formed and absorbed into the body the patient became ill with a high temperature, a rash, and collapse of the circulation. This particular type of tampon was withdrawn, and now the condition is no more common in females than in males.

Staphylococcal food poisoning
Some staphylococci form toxins that cause severe vomiting. If food that has been contaminated with the toxin is eaten, the vomiting comes on after only a few hours and lasts a day or so. Unfortunately these toxins are not destroyed by cooking, but this type of food poisoning, like all others, is prevented by hygiene (handwashing, clean kitchens) and adequate refrigeration of food.

In each of these three diseases the offending types of staphylococci are carried to the patient by fingers and hands. In the case of the scalded skin syndrome this usually means from hospital staff, and in the case of food poisoning from cooks and food handlers.

The three staphylococcal diseases are interesting from the point of view of microbial strategy because the toxins responsible for the diseases seem to be of no benefit to the bacteria. The significance of the toxins lies in the fact that they are at the same time 'superantigens' (see pages 124–125, Chapter 6). This means that they switch on large numbers of T cells at random, whether or not the T cells have anything to do with the immune response to the infection. This interferes with the co-ordination of the response, which is probably useful to the staphylococcal invader. But from the bacteria's point of view there is no point in causing the three diseases mentioned; they are unfortunate side-effects of the superantigen molecule.

THE MICROBE ON ITS OWN DOES THE DAMAGE

It was 1954, and I was investigating tropical fevers in Entebbe, Uganda. One afternoon I came home early from the laboratory feeling ill, with backache, headache, and a temperature of 103°F. By the evening it was worse, and I was taken to the local hospital. It was not malaria, influenza, or a bacterial infection, and although I had been handling yellow fever this was not the culprit. Even in my delirious state I could understand that something very unpleasant was going on inside me, because when a blood sample was taken and injected into laboratory mice, they all died within 36 hours. My blood had this alarming effect even when diluted one part in a million. The illness gradually subsided, but it was a lengthy convalescence, leaving me weak for several months.

The disease was due to Rift Valley Fever virus, an infection that causes epidemics in Eastern and Southern Africa and as far north as Egypt, and which is carried by mosquitoes. Cattle are infected, but the disease is especially severe in sheep. Pregnant ewes abort and most of them die with severe liver damage. Human cases occur and are sometimes fatal, but I had made prodigious quantities of antibody to the virus and got off lightly. There was no epidemic in East Africa at the time, so how did I get infected?

I had accidentally infected myself in the laboratory! While taking blood from an infected mouse an invisible amount of blood had found its way into a badly covered cut on my thumb. Laboratory accidents with microbes such as tuberculosis and hepatitis virus have always been a hazard, and Rift Valley Fever is especially dangerous because such enormous amounts of the virus are present in an infected animal – ten thousand million infectious doses per millilitre of blood.

I mention this personal mishap because in laboratory mice Rift Valley Fever virus is a supreme destroyer of cells. The direct damage is of such a magnitude that this susceptible host may die a mere *six hours after being infected*! This happens when a large dose of the virus is introduced into a mouse's vein. From the blood it passes straight into liver cells, infects nearly all of them, and as soon as it has completed its cycle of growth the liver is almost completely destroyed. In this highly artificial situation all the host defences are overwhelmed. The injected virus is at liberty to enter liver cells almost immediately because the macrophages in the liver (see Figure 9) do not hold it back, and there is no time for defences such as interferon and immunity to make any difference. After the virus's catastrophic effect on cells the liver more or less falls to pieces (liver cells can be seen, floating free, in the blood) and the animal dies. It is the summit of virulence.

Poliomyelitis virus provides another less dramatic example where the damage is done by the microbe itself, not by a toxin or by the host's own response. Poliomyelitis virus occasionally spreads from its normal quarters in the throat and intestine into the blood, and then invades the spinal cord and brain. Here it infects the nerve cells that make muscles contract, multiplies in them, and kills them. If enough nerve cells are knocked out the muscles they supply are weakened or paralysed. Seventy years ago, before the days of polio vaccines, paralysed children were a common sight in infectious disease (fever) hospitals. The paralysed muscles were often those in the arm or leg or, more ominously, the ones used for breathing. To treat the patient with 'respiratory' paralysis these hospitals were equipped with cumbersome, box-like contraptions (iron lungs) into which the patient was placed with the head outside and an air-tight seal round the neck. Inside, regular changes in pressure caused the lungs to suck in air, and breathing was maintained. These iron lungs saved many lives, because the breathing muscles often recovered sufficiently for the patient to be weaned from the iron lung and into the outside world again.

THE HOST INJURES ITSELF

Many microbes do little or no direct damage to cells or tissues, and the disease is largely due to the host's own immune and inflammatory response to the infection. In other words the same response that is needed for defence against parasites can damage normal tissues once it is unleashed. Immunity acts as a two-edged sword, and under extreme circumstances can have lethal consequences, as described above for LCM infection of adult mice.

Pathology caused by immune responses (immunopathology) plays a part in a great number of human infections, and a certain amount of host damage seems unavoidable if infection is to be resisted. Immune inflammation means the arrival of phagocytes and lymphocytes at the site of infection, and this entails swelling and pain. It can be severe and it can last a long time, becoming chronic, but it is a vital part of defence. Immune damage well beyond the call of duty, however, takes place when the focused response directed against the invader also reacts with and damages host tissues. This is what happens in autoimmune diseases (see Box 5), and our example here is rheumatic heart disease.

Tuberculosis, leprosy and glandular fever (EB virus infection) provide good examples where immunopathology seems to account for most of the disease.

Tuberculosis

At school John Keats (1795–1821) loved cricket and boxing, and was fascinated by Greek mythology. He became apprenticed to a surgeon-apothecary when he was 15, and in the same year his mother died of tuberculosis (consumption). Four years later he was enrolled at Guy's Hospital, London, satisfying the examiners and becoming an apothecary in 1816. Soon after, Keats' youngest brother Tom became seriously ill with tuberculosis, and in 1818 Keats lovingly nursed him for two months in a small, dark, airless room. He then set off on a strenuous 600 mile walking tour to Scotland, but after becoming too ill and fevered to continue, he came back to nurse Tom, who died at the end of the year.

By now Keats had developed a cough and was suffering more attacks of fever. From his medical training he would have recognized in himself the warning signs of consumption. He mentions only a sore throat, which could possibly have been due to tuberculosis. It must be remembered that at this time there were only occasional suggestions that consumption was contagious, the stethoscope had only just been invented, and actually measuring fever with the thermometer did not come into practice until 1868. The bacterium that causes tuberculosis was not discovered until 1882.

Keats was also permanently plagued with financial difficulties, and furthermore was unhappy in his love life. His poems refer to weariness, fever, paleness, 'being spectre-thin', all of which are signs of consumption, and also to the wish for 'easeful death'. In spite of these mental and physical stresses some of his greatest works were written between 1818 and 1819. Could it be that the physical disease and stresses were needed for the full flowering of his creative imagination?

After a rushed visit to America in 1819 he was once more unwell, and by

February 1820 had become emaciated and seriously ill. He coughed blood on February 23, and again in June. He looked at the bright red stain on his pillow and said 'I know the colour of that blood. It is arterial blood...that blood is my death warrant.' The diagnosis was obviously pulmonary tuberculosis. He was too ill to write and was nursed by the poet Leigh Hunt and by other friends. As he became weaker and more ill, and in a last desperate bid for recovery, declaring that another winter in London would kill him, he sailed for Italy with his friend the painter Joseph Severn. It was a terrible journey, with storms, sea water in the cabin, bad food, and finally ten days' quarantine of the boat in the Bay of Naples because it was suspected of carrying typhus. On disembarking there was an uncomfortable 138 mile cart-ride from Naples to Rome, taking eight days. They arrived in November 1820, and Severn looked after Keats, who was now much weaker. He vomited two cupfuls of blood on two successive days. Keats described his condition in capital letters as WRETCHED, adding 'when will this posthumous life of mine finish?' He died on February 23, 1821, aged 25, and at the postmortem the lungs were found to be 'entirely destroyed'.

Like most people in the 19th century Keats was surrounded by tuberculosis. In towns and cities it was a universal infection, like the measles. You couldn't avoid it. It is a common theme in Victorian novels, and famous people who have died of it include D.H. Lawrence, Emily Bronte, Anton Chekov, Edgar Allen Poe, Lawrence Sterne, Walter Scott, George Orwell and Vivien Leigh. Adolf Hitler is said to have been traumatized when, aged 13, he saw the body of his father who had died suddenly after a massive tuberculous haemorrhage into the lungs. But tuberculosis was a disease of common people as well as of writers and artists. Ever since 1680, when John Bunyan used the phrase, consumption had been referred to as 'The captain of the men of death'.

Underlying facts

The disease is due to a hardy, waxy, bacterium (*Mycobacterium tuberculosis*) with the ability to invade many different parts of the body. The lung is the commonest organ, and infection takes place by inhaling a bacterium from someone else's lungs; tuberculosis is a disease caught by inspiration! A single cough (or talking for five minutes!) sprays out about 3000 infectious droplets. The inhaled bacterium is deposited in an alveolus (the tiny terminal airspace of the lung) where it is taken up by a resident macrophage (see Figure 9). It is in the macrophage that the decisive battle between parasite and host will eventually be waged. The bacteria grow very slowly, dividing once every day or two compared with once every 20–30 minutes for most bacteria, and they do not form any toxins. But many macrophages die.

The infected individual, unaware of these momentous events, starts an immune response, and if he is lucky it is a good cell-mediated immunity (CMI) response. Antibodies are no use against this invader; what matters is a T cell response, the sort that can switch on and arm the macrophages (see Chapter 3). This takes about a month, during which time the bacteria continue to multiply inside the macrophages. When CMI is finally set in motion, macrophages swarm into the area of infection, phagocytose the bacteria and now begin to kill them.

Often the bacteria enter the body through the throat, and a swelling appears in the neck as the battle rages in the local lymph glands (see Box 28). Swollen glands in the neck were especially common in children drinking unpasteurized milk from cows that were infected with the bovine variety of tuberculosis. I still have a visible swelling in my neck as a result of infection in the 1920s.

All this immune activity takes a month or two, during which the person may have felt slightly off colour or lost some weight because of the cytokines (see Glossary) released into the body by the labouring macrophages.

If all goes well, as it does in nine out of ten infected people, the multiplying bacteria, which have reached the local lymph nodes, are gradually eliminated. What is left is a small island of inflammation and immune cells, just detectable on the X-ray, and the person is now immune to tuberculosis. The immunity can be demonstrated by what is called a *tuberculin test*. Substances from the bacteria are introduced into the skin of the forearm by injection or by placing a pad on the skin (patch test) through which they are absorbed. After 24–48 hours, if the person is immune, the skin goes slightly red because of inflammation and also swollen as immune cells accumulate round the test site.

Not everyone is fortunate enough to respond so successfully. Unless host defences are equal to the task, the island of infection enlarges, and further damage takes place as the immune system struggles to control bacterial growth. A small abscess is formed, containing a cheesy sort of pus and consisting of bacteria and macrophages, some dead some alive, still locked in their struggle. The small swelling, or tubercle (Latin, *tuber* = swelling), is the origin of the word tuberculosis. The bacteria release no toxins, and most of the damage is due to the patient's own CMI response.

At this stage the person feels washed out, develops a cough and is feverish, like John Keats. The infected area gradually enlarges, and a cavity is formed inside it. Once it spreads into a bronchial tube the bacteria can be coughed up and the patient is now infectious for others. Old byelaws against spitting in public originate from the threat of tuberculosis. About half of the

Box 28 Scrofula

During the reign of Charles II (1660–1682) thousands of parents brought their sick children to be 'touched' and cured by the King. The children were suffering from scrofula, which is a type of tuberculosis known for thousands of years. They were unwell, with swollen lymph glands in the neck. Charles II is registered as having touched a total of 92,102 sufferers! From the middle-ages it had been believed that the Royal Houses of England and France had the supernatural gift of curing scrofula in this way, and the popular name for the disease was the Kings Evil. Edward the Confessor (1042–1066) and Clovis of France (481–511) had been famous practitioners. The ceremony included the laying of a 'touchpiece' of gold on the sufferer, to the accompaniment of prayers from the court chaplain. Edward I (1272–1307) touched 533 in a single month and Philip VI of Valois (1328–1350) touched 1500 in a single ceremony. The sheer scale of it rivals that of the hand shaking duties of 20th century royalty. The custom continued until the Stuarts, and Samuel Johnson was one of the last to be touched, by Queen Anne (1702–1714) when he was four years old.

Did it work? Being touched by the King must have given a great boost to the sick child's morale, and not devoid of beneficial effect (see Placebo effect in Glossary). Luckily tuberculosis in the throat and neck more often than not gets better on its own, so that any treatment would have seemed effective. Indeed the Royals might equally well have established a reputation for predicting the sex of unborn children, being correct in 50% of cases.

This type of tuberculosis used to result from drinking milk from cows infected with their strain of tuberculosis. It was controlled by getting rid of infected cows and by pasteurizing milk. At an early stage of the infection the bacteria are carried to local lymph nodes in the neck or intestine, and there, inside macrophages, the struggle to overcome the invader takes place.

people that become ill are infectious for others. If an artery is eroded, bright red blood is coughed up (Keats), sometimes in terrifying quantities, and haemorrhage into the lungs can be fatal (Hitler's father). In addition to cough and fever the patient will by now have lost a lot of weight, the flesh slowly falling away from the bones. Hence old words for tuberculosis include 'phthisis' (wasting) and 'consumption' (being consumed, wasting away). The illness progresses slowly, however, and generally takes years to kill the patient.

Even when you recover from the disease, the tuberculosis bacteria are experts at hanging on. Very occasional survivors remain in the body, tucked away in macrophages, and later in life, if CMI defences are waning, these bacteria begin to multiply and can once more cause disease and spread to other people, as described on page 130.

Those especially vulnerable are small children, those with AIDS because of their depressed CMI, and also people from Africa and India, probably because their genes confer poor CMI responses to tuberculosis (see pages 84–85). In other words, tuberculosis does cause a certain amount of damage on its own, for instance by killing macrophages and releasing their powerful enzymes, even when CMI responses are minimal.

The treatment of tuberculosis was originally by rest, for both the body and mind. For the well-off this was provided in sanatoria, as described in Thomas Mann's novel *The Magic Mountain*. The actual part of the lung that was diseased and had a cavity in it, could be rested by collapsing it by various means so that it no longer took part in breathing. A dramatic change in treatment came in 1946 with discovery of the anti-tuberculosis drug streptomycin. George Orwell was one of the first to be given this drug.

It has been estimated that about a third of the world's population has been infected by tuberculosis, and in the past 200 years it has caused about a thousand million deaths. The big problems with its control are firstly that because the bacteria are often resistant to a drug several drugs now have to be given at once. Secondly, that the drugs are expensive, thirdly that they have to be given for many months (not easy when the patients such as the Somalis in Africa are poor nomadic people), and fourthly that AIDS has made so many people highly susceptible.

Tuberculosis has been called the master adaptor. It is ubiquitous and difficult to dislodge from its place in the human species. Doubtless the large number of genes in its repertoire (it has nearly twice as much DNA as the closely related leprosy bacteria) are what enable it to have such adaptive ingenuity.

Leprosy

Father Damien (1840–1889), whose real name was Joseph de Veuster, was a Belgian priest who visited the Sandwich Islands (Hawaii) in 1865. He was greatly moved by the pitiful state of the 600 lepers who had been consigned by government order to the Island of Molokai (sometimes known as the Friendly Island!). He remained there, devoting himself to their spiritual and physical care. He made a point of eating from the same dishes when sharing their humble meals, he often lent his pipe to a leper, and he did not turn away from the cough of a leper when he was hearing confession. Nevertheless, it was not until 12 years later that he himself got the disease, and he died of it after four years.

Underlying facts

Leprosy (see Box 29) is caused by *Mycobacterium lepri*, a bacterium that was discovered by Hansen, a Norwegian, in 1873. Leprosy was then common in Norway, presumably introduced from infected countries by returning sailors. One of the problems with understanding leprosy has been that the bacteria cannot be cultivated in the laboratory, and for a naturally susceptible animal we have to turn to the armadillo! Luckily the molecular biologists can short-circuit some of these difficulties and, with their ability to sequence DNA and manipulate genes, they are beginning to unravel the mysteries of this microbe.

Leprosy bacteria grow best at the cool temperature found in the skin, in the nerves under the skin, and inside the nose. The testicles are cooler than other organs, and indeed are carried in their ridiculously vulnerable pouch outside the body so as to keep them cool. They too are often damaged in leprosy. Leprosy bacteria, like those of tuberculosis, form no toxins. Even when millions of bacteria are circulating in the blood the patients do not feel unwell, although they would with almost any other bacterium. Only 5% of those infected actually develop the disease. The fascination, from the point of view of those interested in the how's and why's of infectious disease, is in the immune response. Broadly speaking there are two types of immune responders, representing the extremes, with a lot of others in between. It is a spectrum.

One type of leprosy patient makes an excellent CMI response to the bacteria, and develops *tuberculoid* leprosy. The affected areas are full of activated macrophages busily destroying the invaders. The bacteria only divide once every 11–13 days, even slower than tuberculosis bacteria, so the disease unfolds in a very leisurely fashion. In such a leisurely fashion that it may be more than five years before there are any signs and symptoms. Nerves under the skin are infected, especially in the hands and feet, and the exuberant immune response causes a good deal of damage to nerves. Sensation in these nerves is lost, and this means that burns and other mechanical injuries take place over the years and gradually destroy fingers and toes. If the outer layers of the eye (another cool zone) are involved it can lead to ulcers on the cornea and eventual blindness. The sight of a blind leper's hands held out for alms is an irresistible one! But the patient remains well and not very infectious.

Box 29 Leprosy

It might be thought that this is another disease of mainly historical interest, since it was known in biblical times, although it was perhaps confused with the harmless scaly skin disease psoriasis (Greek, *lepros* = scaly). The Crusaders, when they returned from their skirmishes in the Holy Land, brought back with them leprosy, trachoma (see Glossary), and the donkey. By the 13th century there were about 200 leper hospitals in England. Such was the fear of this disease that lepers were abandoned, excluded from society, forced to wear a cowbell or clappers to warn of their approach, and (in mediaeval Spain), declared legally dead! It has been pointed out that leprosy is a disease that affects the body of the patient and the mind of the public. For the well-to-do there were leper colonies, called leprosaria, lazar houses, or lazarettos. St Lazarus, the beggar in the New Testament parable (Luke xiv), full of sores, is the patron saint of lepers. They were not allowed in churches, and occasional parish churches in England have squint windows, consisting of thin slits with a view of the altar, so that the leper could participate in the service while standing outside, unseen by the congregation.

Ten years ago there were more than five million lepers in the world, disabled by the disease, mostly in countries like Africa, India, Latin America and the Pacific Islands, that cannot afford modern drugs, and a large proportion of them were untreated. The number has now fallen to less than a million, and a brand new vaccine is being used. As is so often the case, poverty has a lot to do with susceptibility, and leprosy seems to have retreated from Europe as socioeconomic conditions (crowding, hygiene) have improved.

In the other type of leprosy patient (*lepromatous* leprosy) plenty of antibodies are formed, but there is hardly a flicker of CMI. As we saw with tuberculosis, antibodies are useless, and in a person of this sort the bacteria are able to multiply unrestrainedly. They grow in the nasal mucosa and are expelled in vast numbers with each sneeze or noseblow, so that the patient is very infectious. The skin of the nose, ears and face becomes little short of a living culture chamber for the bacteria (a staggering total of 100,000,000,000 bacteria per patient!) and apart from awesome thickening of the affected skin next to no damage is done. Bacteria also grow in nerves under the skin, but less damage is done than in the tuberculoid form. In infected skin areas there are swarms of bacteria with an occasional macrophage standing by, helpless, having received no invigorating messages from T cells (see Chapter 2). The vigorous but useless antibody response causes various unpleasant immune reactions, characteristic of this type of leprosy.

What is it that determines this great divide in immune responsiveness? It looks as if it is partly due to differences in people's MHC genes (see pages 84–85, 129). For instance, in Africans the tuberculoid response predominates, whereas it is less common in whites, Chinese and Japanese.

Glandular fever

This is the third disease where the immune response is the culprit. It is caused by a herpesvirus, EB virus. It grows in salivary glands and in B cells, is excreted in saliva, and in developing countries nearly all children encounter it by the age of ten. The infection passes unnoticed, because this is a well-behaved parasite and knows its place. The child develops immunity, but the virus is not completely eliminated from the body and remains there for life, tucked away in a very occasional B cell. It also keeps a foothold in salivary glands and is present in the saliva of one out of ten healthy adults. This has been the EB virus pattern throughout most of human history.

In modern 'hygienic' countries, however, where hands, faces, cups and spoons, etc., are regularly washed (and where perhaps there is less family kissing!), children often escape infection. The next opportunity comes after puberty when sexual kissing, especially deep kissing with its salivary exchanges, allows infection. At this stage of life the CMI response is much more vigorous and has unpleasant consequences, and the story of Benjamin was told on page 81.

The virus infects B cells, which are not damaged but are stimulated to produce all sorts of irrelevant antibodies, which are used by the laboratory in diagnosis. The T cells, however, respond immunologically to the infected B cells and try to eliminate them, as described in Part 3. The result is an immunological civil war. The person feels ill because of the release of cytokines, and develops swelling of the spleen, lymph nodes and tonsils, where the battle is being fought. The disease, glandular fever, with a severe sore throat, malaise and swollen glands, can linger on for months before the T cells gain the upper hand. Even then the virus often continues to be excreted in the saliva.

An unnecessary burden of heart disease

In many developing countries the commonest type of heart disease is caused by streptococcal bacteria. What happens is that a child gets a bad sore throat due to a streptococcus, but forms antibody to the bacteria and recovers. Unfortunately in some children the antibody against the bacteria also react with the heart, and a few weeks later gives rise to a disease called rheumatic fever. If this child suffers further sore throats, caused by different varieties of streptococci, more antibodies are formed and the heart damage gets worse. The lucky children who live in the developed world are given penicillin, which will also prevent further infections by streptococci, and therefore this sort of heart disease is a rarity. But in many developing countries streptococcal sore throats go untreated, unprevented, and in 1999 there were a tragic 30 million children with this type of heart disease. Three-quarters of them will die prematurely, at an average age of 35.

THE MICROBE CAUSES CANCER AS A LATE EFFECT

Sometimes the damage done by a microbe takes many years to become apparent. It is not too difficult to make the connection between streptococcal infection and rheumatic fever because the latter appears a few weeks after the former. Antibodies formed against the streptococci react also with the heart and cause damage (myocarditis). The repeated streptococcal attacks that result in permanent damage to the heart can be prevented by antibiotics, but for three-quarters of the world's population rheumatic heart disease is still common – commonest of all in Aborigines in the Northern Territory of Australia.

When the result of infection is not seen for ten years (in other words when there is an incubation period of ten years) it is much more difficult to make the connection. The disease SSPE (subacute sclerosing panencephalitis, see Glossary) may not come on for ten years or so after measles, and the disease kuru has been recorded more than 15 years after cannibalistic eating of infected human organs (see pages 202–206). An incubation period as long as this is now an accepted part of our outlook, but when it was first proposed our minds had to take a quantum jump before accepting it.

Now we think nothing of suggesting, for instance, that multiple sclerosis or rheumatoid arthritis is a very late consequence of infection. Many would have been glad to find that cancers were caused by microbes, because it would mean that a vaccine to prevent the infection would also prevent the cancer. Alas, there are only a few microbes firmly associated with cancers and even then the actual way in which they do it is unknown.

Certain cancers, however, are due to the delayed action of viruses, and sometimes the evidence is convincing. The virus is present in the cancer cells, where it is the subtle effects on cell divisions that cause cancer. But extra factors (cofactors) are probably needed. Not everyone who is infected gets the cancer.

Hepatitis B and liver cancer

Joseph Mbule, aged 34, lives in a small village in the Gambia, West Africa. He is normally quite healthy, but has not been feeling well for some weeks, occasionally feverish, and his wife has noticed he is getting thinner, although the same can not be said for his stomach. And now, for the last day or two, there is this pain on the right side of his stomach, just below the ribs. It is time to make the bicycle journey to the clinic. The doctor examines him, finds that the liver is considerably enlarged, and takes him straight into hospital. The outlook is gloomy because liver cancer is so common in this part of Africa, and the weight loss, fever and swelling of the stomach are typical symptoms. Joseph's cousin died from it only last year.

Tests showed that it was indeed cancer of the liver and not cancer of another organ with deposits in the liver. As Joseph and his family heard the bad news they remembered that his cousin had only survived for three months after the diagnosis had been made.

Underlying facts
Hepatitis (inflammation of the liver) can be caused by seven different viruses, which are labelled alphabetically (see Box 30). They all grow in the liver and cause hepatitis.

Joseph, when he was a small child, had been infected with hepatitis B. It didn't make him ill, because the virus itself doesn't do any direct harm. The damage is not done until T cells start killing off the infected cells, and children make a poor immune response to this infection. It is an example of immunopathology (see pages 167–168). But his poor immune response also allowed the virus to stay in his liver and blood. When the virus infects adults, on the other hand, they make a good immune response, which goes with a more severe illness but eventual elimination of the virus from the body.

Joseph became a healthy 'carrier' of hepatitis B virus, and stayed that way, capable of infecting other people. Like many others in the Gambia he had

---

Box 30 The hepatitis alphabet

Hepatitis B — this virus was encountered accidentally by an American anthropologist, Baruch Blumberg, who found a new protein (antigen) in the serum of Australian Aborigines, and called it 'Australia antigen'. This later turned out to be a protein from a new virus (hepatitis B), and the anthropologist was awarded the Nobel Prize for his discovery. After infection and recovery from the acute hepatitis B illness one in ten people fail to eliminate the virus, which stays in the liver and blood for many years. The person is quite well but is a carrier. The earlier in life you are infected the more likely it is that you will become a carrier. Mothers easily infect their children, and the virus is also spread by contaminated needles and syringes (drug abuse, tattooing, ear-piercing, acupuncture). Blood is tested before being used for transfusion.

Our understanding of hepatitis B has been helped by the fact that very similar viruses are found in woodchucks, ground squirrels, Peking ducks and kangaroos. Animals that become virus carriers tend to get liver cancer.

The rest of the alphabet

Hepatitis A — spreads by the faecal–oral method, and is generally not very severe. Infection is common in parts of the world where hygiene is poor, and at one time people visiting such countries were given an injection of antibody to the virus (gammaglobulin) to protect them, but we now have a first-rate vaccine.

Hepatitis C — not discovered until 1989. It invades the blood, and spreads to other people like hepatitis B. Illness is mild but infection often becomes chronic, the virus staying in the blood for years, and it can cause liver cancer.

Hepatitis E — this is spread by the faecal–oral route, often in water. Not a severe infection but very common in India.

Hepatitis D, Hepatitis F, Hepatitis G — also present in blood and can spread by blood transfusions, etc.

---

acquired the virus from his mother, who was a carrier. In developed countries less than one in a hundred people are carriers, but they are very common in the Gambia and worldwide there are 350 million of them. Nearly all are well, and became infected early in life.

Carriers of hepatitis B virus are 200 times more likely to get liver cancer than non-carriers, and the cancer does not develop until 20–30 years after infection. In Africa it is the commonest cancer in men. But not all carriers get the cancer, so other factors (cofactors) must have an influence. Aflatoxin, a fungal substance present in contaminated peanuts, possibly acts as a cofactor.

There is a good vaccine against hepatitis B, and its large-scale use in infants in the Gambia and in many other countries will prevent infection and thus prevent the cancer. However, once you are a carrier you usually remain one, so for the time being there will be many more like Joseph who succumb to liver cancer.

Genital warts and cervical cancer

Wart viruses are described on page 116. In the cervix, the first sign of infection is not an actual wart but a flat area of infected cells (seen in a cervical smear test). There are many different genital wart viruses, but with two or three of them in particular the infected cells may transform and become cancer cells. It happens only in one or two people per hundred infected, so presumably there are cofactors such as cigarette smoking or infection with a herpesvirus.

In the USA 608 young college women were carefully checked for genital warts every six months for three years. During this time 43% became infected with one of the 16 different genital wart viruses tested for. Each new infection tended to persist, as do the viruses in skin warts, and lasted an average of eight months. The longer the virus stayed, the more likely it was to cause abnormalities in cervical smears.

Leukaemia and viruses

One of the retroviruses (see page 10), only discovered in 1980, is an undoubted cause of the type of leukaemia where T cells are the villains. The virus, Human T cell Leukaemia Virus type 1 (HTLV1), infects T cells and turns them into cancerous (leukaemic) cells. It is quite common in Japan and the West Indies, and spreads between people by way of blood and milk (breastfeeding). The African pygmy chimpanzee, our closest relative, with 98.4% of its DNA identical to ours, has a very similar virus, which is probably the source of our HTLV1.

The mouse retrovirus that causes breast cancer in mice was referred to on page 127, but there is no human equivalent.

EB virus; catching glandular fever in the wrong part of the world

EB virus, which causes glandular fever, is closely linked with a cancer of the nose and throat (nasopharygeal carcinoma) that is common in South China and parts of Asia. The cancer cells all contain the virus, but a cofactor is needed for the tumour to develop, possibly the nitrosamines present in salted fish. EB virus is also linked with Burkitt's lymphoma, a cancer of B cells seen in children in East Africa and Papua New Guinea. Here, too, the cancer cells contain the virus (B cells are the regular host cells), but a cofactor must be necessary (possibly malaria) because the tumour is not seen in children elsewhere in the world infected with this ubiquitous virus.

The story of oncogenes in chicken cancer

Oncogenes, see Box 31, are bad news for chickens but exciting objects for virologists and cancer researchers. Their role in human cancer is not clear.

The immune system and cancer

When a cancer is caused by a virus, then vaccination against infection will prevent the cancer. This is what is happening with the vaccine against hepatitis B virus. Does the immune system protect against the cancer itself? Is this one of its functions? The present state of play is outlined in Box 32.

THE MICROBE STAYS FOREVER, LYING LOW, OCCASIONALLY VENTURING OUT TO CAUSE TROUBLE

Case history – shingles on a shopkeeper's shoulder

It was a smart men's clothing store, and David Spence had built it up from nothing. He was now 66, slowing down, and was thinking of retiring and handing over the business to his son. One morning, he woke up with a sore right shoulder. It was a burning feeling, yet seemed only skin deep, and he assumed he had been scratching it while he was asleep. He thought nothing more of it. At the end of the day, however, it was worse and the next morning the skin over the back of the shoulder felt as if it was on fire, as if some nasty chemical irritant had been rubbed into it. To his great surprise

---

Box 31 Oncogenes and cancer

Oncogenes (Greek, *onkos* = swelling, tumour) are genes present in normal cells, whose job is to control cell division and cell behaviour. There are at least 20 of them, and when they misbehave, having been inappropriately stimulated, the cell breaks free from its normal restraints, multiplies, and spreads through the body. The patient now has a malignant cancer.

Oncogenes can be switched on by some chemicals, and certain types of retrovirus (though not HIV) have their own oncogenes. These oncogenes were acquired from host cells in the remote past, but are of no use to the virus. When such a virus infects a cell it turns it into a cancer cell. In 1966, aged 87, Dr Peyton Rous was awarded the Nobel Prize for discovering, 55 years earlier, that certain chicken cancers were due to retroviruses, the cancers spreading through the flock like an infectious disease. But nothing of this sort happens in humans, and the role of oncogenes in human cancer is still uncertain.

---

his wife said she could see nothing there except two very small red spots. The next day the pain was worse still, especially when he stood under the shower and used the towel. If anything he was slightly off colour, but was able to carry on working in the shop, and the pain was helped by parac-etamol. This continued for a week, the area of burning pain spreading round to the right side of the chest, and one or two more red spots appeared, start-ing as little blisters before scabbing over. It gradually got better, but a month later, retired and otherwise well, he still had occasional twinges. It was three months before the shoulder felt completely normal.

Underlying facts

The shopkeeper had suffered a mild attack of shingles (zoster). It is due to the same virus that causes chickenpox, and the story is much the same as with the cold sore virus (herpes simplex) as described on pages 93–95, Chapter 5. Nearly all of us catch chickenpox during childhood. Chickenpox, by the way, does not refer to the bird...the word chicken was used in olden days to refer to a child. The chickenpox virus spreads through the body by way of the blood and reaches the skin where it grows to form virus-rich blisters. The illness is a very mild one, often not recognized by the mother, and the child recovers and the immune response eliminates the virus. But not entirely. As in the case of the cold sore, the virus has by now migrated

Box 32 Does the immune system protect us against cancer?

Cancer cells can be thought of as parasites, no longer under the body's control. They break loose, spreading and multiplying as if they were foreign invaders. In their ruthless pursuit of immortality they eventually kill the host.

Many types of cancer cell have acquired surface antigens that are foreign to the body. Immune responses would be expected against those cancerous antigens, and the cancer cells should be eliminated, for instance by cytotoxic T cells (see Chapter 3). But cancer cells escape this fate and continue to divide. This is sometimes because they reduce the number of MHC molecules displayed on their surface so that T cells cannot recognize them (see Box 8), or because they secrete substances that suppress the immune system. For example, cancers of the prostate, breast, kidney, lung and ovary produce a certain cytokine (TGF beta) that interferes with the immune response. The patient with cancer is then powerless.

It is possible that isolated cancer cells arise quite frequently in most of us and are recognized and killed by the immune system, although some are harder to recognize and kill than others. So what is it that makes some people develop a full-blown, life-threatening cancer? Evidently the immune system is only one part of it, because in people with a depressed immune system, for instance after a kidney transplant, it is only one or two special types of cancer that become more common. There is no general flowering of cancers in these patients.

Nevertheless, immunological approaches to treatment sound promising. For instance, the patient's cancer cells, treated so as not to divide, can be injected so as to act as a vaccine against the cancer (see pages 239–245, Chapter 11). Or an antibody formed against the cancer cells could be 'armed' by joining onto it a killer substance like ricin (once used on the end of a pointed walking stick by a KGB agent to kill a Bulgarian diplomat), so that when the antibody docks on its cancer cell target it delivers a lethal hit. Or the patient's T cells, handicapped by the cancer, could be removed, stimulated and increased in number in the test tube, then reinjected into the patient to boost the immune response. Alternatively the immune system could be given a more rough and ready stimulation by injecting Bacillus Calmettte–Guérin (BCG – see Glossary) or cytokines. Each of these approaches has been tried out in the laboratory but none is yet suitable for routine use.

up local sensory nerves (Figure 18) and entered nerve cells in the ganglia that lie along the spine or at the base of the skull, depending on where the chickenpox spots are. Once in the nerve cells it does not multiply or release any antigens. Securely entrenched and in latent form it lies low, waiting its opportunity.

As the person gets older, and increasingly so after the age of 60, CMI to this particular virus weakens. One day the virus comes to life again in a nerve cell in one of the ganglia. It spreads to neighbouring cells, which are stimulated by this activity, sending off messages to the brain, and the person feels itching or pain in the area of skin supplied by that particular ganglion (one shoulder and one side of the chest in the shopkeeper). The virus meanwhile is spreading down nerves to the same area of skin, where it multiplies, and in a few days the blistery spots of shingles appear. As spots they are exactly the same as in the original chickenpox, and they are infectious for any non-immune children in the vicinity. Also for any adults unlucky enough to have escaped chickenpox during childhood,

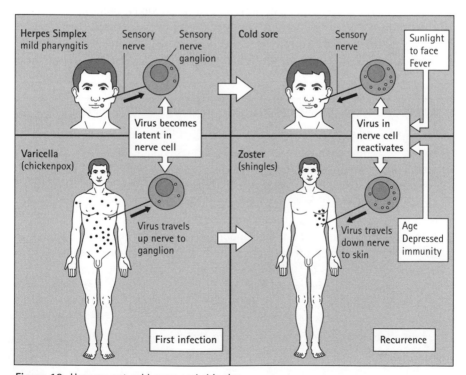

Figure 18 How we get cold sores and shingles.

who may now suffer a more troublesome disease. It often takes a long time for lymphocytes and macrophages to clear up the infection in the ganglion, and for the nerve cells to settle down. This means that the pain can continue for weeks or months. If the face and the eye are affected it can be a very unpleasant illness, and treatment with the new drug ganciclovir is helpful.

The shopkeeper's shingles, therefore, was caused by the chickenpox virus that had taken up residence in his nerve ganglia, and it re-emerged onto the skin 60 years later in fully infectious form. Shingles thus originates from inside the body – you don't catch it from someone else. Because it arises in a single ganglion it involves only the area of skin supplied by that ganglion, and it is only on one side of the body.

This is the strategy by which the virus has maintained itself in its human host over the generations for tens of thousands of years, as explained in Box 33. But perhaps not for much longer, as far as chickenpox virus goes. There are ominous signs in the shape of a vaccine that protects children from infection and this vaccine could unseat the virus from its place in our species.

Several microbes are experts at hanging on in the body, making a mockery of the immune responses that are supposed to eliminate them. They *persist*. This way of life comes naturally to many viruses, which hide in the infected cell for an indefinite period, and without multiplying or betraying their

---

Box 33 Staying on; why persistence pays and latency matters

Throughout 99.9% of our history we have lived in small groups of up to a few score people. A microbe that infects the individual, spreads to infect others in the group, and is then eliminated from the body by the immune response, is unlikely to survive under these circumstances. After infecting all in the group it will have nowhere else to go and will die out, unless it is so tough (having resistant spores or cysts) that it can keep alive in the outside world waiting for another opportunity. The only microbes that could have maintained themselves in the human species during those tens of thousands of years before the development of agriculture, the rise of towns and cities and before people became more numerous, were those that came from other animals or from biting insects, or those that stayed on in the body after infection. By staying on in the individual and later reactivating, the microbe could spread to the children and grandchildren and thus stay on in the group. In the example of chickenpox the disease

---

Box 33 Staying on; why persistence pays and latency matters (continued)

kept disappearing from the small community, but periodically re-emerged when the virus reactivated as shingles in an older person, by which time a new crop of uninfected children would have appeared.

It was persistent microbes like this, and presumably the normal flora, both closely adapted to the human host that Ogden Nash (1902–1971) must have had in mind in his poem about the germ:

> 'A mighty creature is the germ
> Though smaller than the pachyderm
> His customary dwelling place
> Is deep within the human race...'

The infections that come to us directly from animals and that don't depend on a chain of human infection include rabies and leptospirosis (see Glossary). Those that come from biting insects include malaria and filariasis (see Glossary). Otherwise, all the current human infections that don't stay on could not have existed 100,000 years ago. They must have arisen after the birth of towns and cities.

We know from studies of measles on different-sized islands that this virus needs a population of at least half a million if it is to maintain itself without being periodically reintroduced from outside. There must at all times be someone actually suffering from measles, and it therefore cannot survive in small groups of people. The same would be true for the common cold, influenza and poliomyelitis.

When small, completely isolated Indian communities in the Amazon basin were first encountered by intrepid scientists they somehow obtained blood samples, which were tested for antibodies to different viruses. The viruses present in these communities were thus identified. There was no poliomyelitis, influenza, measles or mumps, and the only ones present were those that persist (stay on) in the body, such as herpesviruses, wart viruses, adenoviruses and polyomaviruses (see Glossary). Bacterial infections such as typhoid and tuberculosis (see pages 199–201, 168–172) come into the same category.

Persistence has therefore been an immense advantage in microbial evolution. Persistence is not an easy thing for a microbe to achieve. Various sophisticated techniques have been adopted, and the microbe needs to exercise great cunning and self control in its outwitting of immune defences.

presence. The important ones are those that, like chickenpox virus, are capable of coming to life again after a long interval and causing disease. Years after encountering the original infection the person, who has recovered and has remained perfectly well, once more develops a disease and is a source of infection for others. We call this type of persistence *latency*; the virus is latent and can become patent. Viruses in the same category include adenoviruses, wart viruses and polyomaviruses (see Glossary), but the most accomplished practitioners are the herpesviruses. The significance for the virus of this way of life is outlined in Box 33.

Chickenpox virus is a herpesvirus, and there are at least eight different human herpesviruses (see Box 34). They are such successful microbes that they are present in everyone everywhere in the world. As you sit reading this sentence you have most of them in your nerve ganglia, salivary glands, or lymphocytes. We now identify them by numbers, which is useful because new ones are discovered every year or two! Chickenpox–shingles virus is human herpesvirus number 3. Although this one spreads to others from the virus-rich blisters on the skin, most of the herpesviruses spread via saliva, growing in the region of the mouth or in the salivary gland. They have accompanied our species through much of its evolution and have got used to infecting us during childhood.

Most of the non-viral microbes are no good at latency because they release molecules that cause inflammation, but some of the ones that live inside cells (tuberculosis, typhoid, malaria) have mastered the art. The story for typhoid and malaria is told in Chapter 9.

MICROBES AS POSSIBLE CULPRITS IN DIABETES, MULTIPLE SCLEROSIS, RHEUMATOID ARTHRITIS, ETC.

We are still in the dark about the cause of a surprising number of chronic diseases. 'Allergy' and 'viruses' have been popular suggestions, but the evidence is generally poor. Yet it would be of immense importance if a microbe of some sort could be incriminated. There would then be something to focus on, an opportunity to develop a vaccine against the microbe and thus prevent the disease. Likewise, if the disease were due to 'allergy', meaning the patient's own immune response, we could possibly identify the antigen that was causing the response, and inhibit that response.

Because it would be so important to identify a guilty microbe (or immune response), researchers have been, if anything, over-enthusiastic in their hunt, not self-critical enough and the rest of us have been too eager to grasp

---

Box 34 Herpes by numbers

- HHV1 (Human Herpes Virus 1 or herpes simplex virus). This is the cold sore virus, and it usually enters the body by way of a tiny abrasion in the mouth. Its subsequent travels were described on pages 93–95 and Figure 18).
- HHV2. This is a substrain of HHV1 that has successfully adapted itself to the genital areas and thus given rise to a new sexually transmitted disease.

Both HHV 1 and HHV 2 can cause various other, less pleasant conditions, such as meningitis, which are important for the sufferer and for the physician. But not for the virus, because invasion of places like the meninges (the coverings of the brain) is a 'dead end' that does not lead to infection of fresh hosts in the outside world. The virus is only 'interested' in spreading from one person to another and surviving, keeping its position as an ancient human parasite.

- HHV3 (chickenpox/shingles or varicella/zoster virus).
- HHV4 or EB virus. The story of EB virus, which makes its home in the immune system, is given on page 175, Chapter 8.
- HHV5, or cytomegalovirus. Cytomegalovirus should be awarded a prize for being one of the best-behaved human parasites. It grows harmlessly in salivary glands and only causes trouble when our immune defences are wrecked, as in AIDS, or when pregnant women are infected for the first time, because the fetus can then be infected and damaged. Surely then, this is not such a well-behaved virus. But remember that during 99.9% of the time it has been associated with humans it has been accustomed to infecting all children, and there was virtually no chance of it infecting a pregnant woman because she would already be resistant. And individuals with serious immune defects would not have survived anyway.
- HHV6 and HHV7 grow in salivary glands and in T cells, and infect us all by the age of five and then persist in the body, but are harmless apart from causing a very mild feverish illness with a rash.
- HHV8 is a recently discovered member, again present in saliva and persistent. Present in ejaculates of many normal adults, so it probably spreads also via sexual activity. Harmless except that it is somehow associated with a special type of tumour called Kaposi's sarcoma, seen in AIDS patients.

whatever is offered. False alarms, unconfirmed reports, 'breakthroughs', they have come with such regularity that a separate book could be written on this subject!

In Box 35 I have summarized the current state of play for these chronic diseases, with my assessment of how good the evidence is. We have to be fussy about it. It is not enough just to show that, say, a virus is nearly always present in the disease, because the virus may be one of those that stay around in the body anyway, or it may have arrived after the disease started. On the other hand, some of the diseases look very much as if they could be late results of infection, remembering that even with a known infectious disease it may take ten years or so for signs and symptoms to appear, for instance kuru (see pages 202–204), or SSPE as a late result of measles (see Glossary).

The case for a microbe always looks better when it causes a very similar chronic disease in an animal. A certain type of Coxsackie virus (see Glossary) causes diabetes in mice, and hepatitis B-like viruses cause liver cancer in various animals. It would be easy to nail the microbe if everyone who was infected got the disease. Unfortunately this does not seem to be the case. You may have to have certain genes (see pages 84–85) if you are to make the sort of immune response to the microbe that starts off the disease, or you may need to be a smoker, or conceivably an eater of a certain food item. Demonstrating that a microbe causes an uncommon disease can be difficult when nearly everyone carries that microbe, just as it would have been hard to prove that smoking causes lung cancer if everyone smoked.

But the hunt continues. We have amazingly sensitive molecular methods, and can pick up a single molecule of a microbe's DNA. Perhaps new human viruses will be discovered and incriminated. And meanwhile, when we think of infectious agents causing these diseases, we should remind ourselves that, as was said of the existence of life elsewhere in the universe, 'Absence of evidence is not evidence of absence.'

Box 35 Do microbes cause these chronic diseases?

Disease	Suggested microbes	Quality of evidence
Diabetes (the sort that starts early in life and needs insulin)*	Coxsackie virus (see Glossary)	Quite good, for some cases only
Inflammatory bowel disease (Crohn's disease, ulcerative colitis)*	Viruses, e.g. measles; certain bacteria	Very poor
Multiple sclerosis**	Viruses (at least eight different ones suggested)	Fair, no single virus involved
Rheumatoid arthritis* (not osteoarthritis)	Viruses (EB virus, rubella) Bacteria	Poor
Peptic ulcer	Bacteria (Helicobacter pylori)	Very good (see Box 12)
Ankylosing spondylitis (chronic arthritis of the spine)*	Bacteria (Klebsiella, see Glossary)	Good
Chronic fatigue syndrome (myalgic encephalo-myelitis or ME)	Viruses (EB virus and others)	Not good; viruses may cause some cases
Alzheimer's disease	'Virus'	No evidence
Heart attacks	Coxsackie virus	Good, in a minority of cases
Cancer (cervical and liver cancer, certain leukemias, etc.)	see pages 176–180, Chapter 8	Good

* Diseases where the immune response plays an important part. ** An estimated two-and-a-half million people in the world have multiple sclerosis, 85,000 of them in the UK.

Chapter 9

THUMBNAIL SKETCHES OF SEVEN SELECTED DISEASES

In a book like this it is impossible to deal with all human infections. Here, I want to tell you about seven infectious diseases, selected for their general interest and because they show the successes and failures of the immune defences described in Chapter 3.

SYPHILIS AND CIVILIZATION

Portrait of a Renaissance man

Girolamo Fracastoro (1483–1553) came from Verona and was a man of wide interests, excelling in both the arts and the sciences. He wrote a book on astronomy, foreshadowing some of the discoveries of his fellow-student in Padua, the great astronomer Nicolaus Copernicus. He also struggled with the problem of attraction and repulsion between bodies, a problem solved in later years by Newton, and he was the first to suggest the use of rectolinear maps and use the word 'pole' for the ends of the earth's axis. His Latin poetry was of the highest quality, and his relevance in the book you are now reading is that he wrote an epic Latin poem called 'Syphilis, sive Morbus Gallicus' (syphilis or the French disease), completed in 1530. Syphilis had arrived in Europe in 1493.

In the poem a shepherd called Syphilus is afflicted with the disease that was called after him. The incubation period is described in colourful terms:

> *'The disease, in fact, does not show itself at once by*
> *accusing symptoms directly that it has penetrated the*

> *organism. For a certain time it broods in silence, as if it were gathering its forces for a more terrible explosion.'*

The symptoms are then portrayed:

> *'Syphilus...manifested the foul sores in his own body; first he knew sleepless nights, his bones ached mercilessly.'*

Treatments are referred to, which included mercury and guaiacum (the juice of a certain tree).

Fracastoro's other great medical work *De Contagione* (1546) contains a remarkable statement of modern ideas about the nature of infection. At that time diseases were generally attributed to miasmas (mists) or the planets. He proposed that infections were transmitted as seeds (seminaria) in three ways. First by contact, passing like the seeds of putrefaction 'from one cluster of grapes to another'. Second, indirectly, by materials such as clothes and linen:

> *'It is, indeed, wonderful how the infection of phthisis or pestilential fevers may cling to bedding clothes.'*

Third, transfer at a distance (as well as by direct contact). He gives smallpox and phthisis (tuberculosis) as examples, and we now count this as airborne droplet.

Underlying facts

Syphilis is caused by the bacterium *Treponema pallidum* (Latin = pale corkscrew), so-called because it has a spiral shape and is pale in the sense that it is not easily stained for microscopic observation. It is an ancient disease, with a rich and interesting history.

The bacteria are transmitted during sexual intercourse and enter the body through tiny breaks in the skin or mucous membranes. They divide only every 30 hours, but spread to local lymph nodes and reach the blood at an early stage. About three weeks later (Fracastoro's incubation period), when the number of bacteria at the site of infection has increased to at least ten million and hordes of immune cells have arrived there, a hard but painless lump develops. This is called the *primary chancre*. Lymph nodes in the groin are now enlarged.

The skin overlying the chancre soon breaks down, and if a tiny drop of liquid is taken from it and examined under the microscope the bacteria can be identified and the diagnosis made. Unfortunately these bacteria, like those of leprosy, cannot be cultivated except in laboratory animals. At this stage the infected person feels alright, but the bacteria in the blood are invading the liver, the joints and the skin and mucous membranes elsewhere in the body. After a month or two he feels unwell, with fever and muscle aches and pains. In the poem his (Syphilus') bones 'ached mercilessly'. Spots and ulcers appear on the skin and mucous membranes, and these are teeming with bacteria. If the patient is female and unlucky enough to be pregnant the bacteria invade the placenta, reach the fetus, which is often born suffering from congenital syphilis. The picture of the congenitally infected child is a classical one, although it is now less common than it used to be. At least 100,000 of the 12 million new cases of syphilis in the world in 1996 would have been congenital.

The immune system is doing its best. Antibodies are formed, cell-mediated immunity (CMI) becomes detectable, and the number of bacteria is greatly reduced. The patient is now no longer infectious, but often a few bacteria stay on in the body and avoid destruction. The immune system makes heroic attempts to deal with these hangers on, which are mostly in the brain, bones, heart and aorta. But the constant immune onslaught causes gradual damage and destruction in these organs, and the patient eventually, up to 20 years after being infected, suffers heart failure and neurological disease. The latter may include muscle paralysis and loss of intellect ('general paralysis of the insane').

Syphilis is a major debilitating, disfiguring disease, but only kills about one in ten of those infected, and only if they remain untreated. The first real advance in treatment was when Paul Ehrlich discovered that arsenic (in the form of Salvarsan) was helpful. The breakthrough came when penicillin was discovered and this is still the best drug.

Syphilis is now much less common than it used to be, thanks to penicillin and the tracing and treating of sexual contacts. The tracing of contacts is made easier because the incubation period between getting infected and developing the ability to infect others is a month or so. Therefore contacts can often be located and treated before they have had time to pass on the bacteria to others. Gonorrhoea, in contrast, has an incubation period of only 2–7 days. When a patient has gonorrhoea the people he or she infects will be able to pass it on to others within a week, before they can be traced and treated. One amazing example of the follow up of syphilis contacts was a prostitute in Los Angeles who in 1970 developed syphilis. She kept a diary of all her customers, mostly truck drivers, together with their home addresses (!), and there had been 310 over the course of the past 4–5 months. They were resident in 38 different States, yet 168 of them were tracked down.

Seven were found to have syphilis and were treated; they had not infected their wives.

Like other sexually transmitted diseases, syphilis is commonest at the peak of sexual activity (15–30 years), and special at-risk groups include long-distance lorry drivers, seamen, male homosexuals, and tourists. As with the other sexually transmitted diseases it can be prevented by condoms, which have been shown to hold back microbes in the following type of test. Different viruses (herpes simplex, HIV) or bacteria (syphilis, gonorrhoea) were introduced into a condom, which was then fitted over the end of a suitable sized syringe plunger, as a fake penis. After fake coitus (moving the contraption around in sterile fluid for about half an hour) the surrounding fluid was tested and found free of infection. In some of the tests it was left in the sterile fluid for a further (surely excessive) eight hours. The world's condom requirements are astronomical. Each year 500–800 million are imported by donor agencies into African, Caribbean and Pacific zones. Half of them are made in the USA, and more people are employed testing them than making them. At present there is only one condom-manufacturing plant in Africa.

It may be noted that in syphilis, as with other sexually transmitted diseases, the necessary instrument of transmission is the penis. When this is missing, as in female homosexuals, who are also less promiscuous, these infections are uncommon. Promiscuity, needless to say, is not a new thing. The well-charted sexual adventures of Casanova (1725–1798) brought him a harvest that included four attacks of gonorrhoea (see Glossary) and one of syphilis, while James Boswell (1740–1795) on his evening excursions in London, experienced no less than 19 episodes of urethritis (mainly gonococcal).

Most people believe syphilis was carried to Europe by Columbus' sailors when they came back to Spain from the New World in 1493. It arrived in Scotland in 1496 with Charles VIII of France's mercenaries, who had come to help Peter Warbeck (pretender to the English throne) invade England. The sexual connection was well recognized and in April 1497 the Burgh of Aberdeen called for all loose women to 'decist fra ther vicis and syne of venerie' and work for their support, on pain of being branded. But all attempts to prevent it spreading failed and the new disease was well established throughout Europe five years after it had arrived. It was a serious, life-threatening disease, and its impact was comparable to that of AIDS today.

If syphilis was brought to Europe by the sailors of Christopher Columbus, what was its history before then? The answers, still uncertain, are outlined in Box 36.

Box 36 The origins of syphilis

In its present form neither syphilis, nor indeed any of the sexually transmitted diseases, could have maintained itself in prehistoric times (see Box 33). There are, however, some closely related bacteria that could have done so and which are probably the microbial ancestors of syphilis. The disease Yaws is seen in tropical and subtropical countries and is due to *Treponema pertenue*, very similar to *T. pallidum*. Ulcers and open sores are formed on the body surface, full of bacteria, and the infection spreads by direct contact, especially in children. Years later the healed sores may break down, so that the person once more becomes infectious. It seems quite likely that about 6000 years ago, in parts of the world where humans began to congregate into towns and cities (e.g. Mesopotamia), the yaws-type bacteria faced local extinction because people were wearing clothing, and transfer from skin to skin was now becoming more difficult. But the bacteria were ideally fitted for the new conditions if they spread by the sexual route; clothing if anything encourages rather than interferes with sexual activity and multiple sexual partners were more likely in crowded communities. Thus modern syphilis arose, perhaps about 3000 years ago. According to this view it has been in Europe for a long time, although it may in the 15th century have changed to a more serious disease (it was referred to as the '*great* pox', worse than the *small*pox). So perhaps Christopher Columbus did not bring it back from America. Like many other adventurers and explorers, he doubtless gave more than he acquired, from a microbiological point of view.

Shakespeare refers to syphilis (e.g. Timor's speech, Act 3, scene 3, *Troilus and Cressida*) as well as to gonorrhoea, but later writers generally steered clear of the subject of sexually transmitted diseases. It was not until 1881 that Ibsen's play, *Ghosts*, gave a shattering portrayal of syphilis to a startled world. Nevertheless it was a common disease, and sufferers too numerous to mention included popes, kings, artists, writers and composers, as well as countless common mortals.

For a while, syphilis was confused with gonorrhoea (see Glossary). In 1767 the British surgeon John Hunter (1728–1793) inoculated his own penis with pus from a patient with gonorrhoea. Unfortunately the patient had syphilis as well as gonorrhoea and the intrepid investigator developed both diseases. He therefore decided the two must be the same. Although Jean Francois Hernandez in 1812 inoculated convicts in Toulon with gonorrhoeal pus without producing syphilis, the two were not finally separated until 1879, when Albert Neisser discovered the bacterium that causes gonorrhoea (*Neisseria gonorrhoeae*, or the gonococcus). Today,

> **Box 36 The origins of syphilis (continued)**
>
> although we know the entire DNA 'bar code' of syphilis, with its 1000 or
> so genes, we are woefully ignorant about its life inside infected people.
> Perhaps, like smallpox, the disease will be eliminated from the earth
> before we have unravelled its secrets.'

MEASLES AND ITS INVASION PLAN

The English Hippocrates

Thomas Sydenham (1624–1689) went to Oxford to read medicine, but his studies were interrupted when he joined Cromwell's army. He was commissioned as a Captain of Cavalry and took part in fierce fighting. He returned to Oxford in 1646 after being wounded, and was awarded his Bachelor of Medicine degree in 1648. After studies in Montpellier, France, his final degree of Doctor of Medicine was from Cambridge in 1676, and he settled into practice in London.

As a physician Sydenham relied on careful examination of the patient and he kept meticulous records. This was a time when most physicians were happy to diagnose the disease and prescribe treatment by mere examination of a urine sample – there was no need to see the patient!

Sydenham gave good descriptions of gout (he suffered from it), of chorea (a convulsive disease of children known as St Vitus Dance) and of syphilis. He also distinguished between the fevers of malaria (tertian ague), dysentery (the bloody flux), typhoid (enteric fever) and typhus (see Glossary).

Which brings us to measles. Since the middle ages measles had been regarded as a mild form of smallpox, but, Sydenham's description of the disease, in Latin, was unmistakable. He gives a day by day account. The preliminary common cold-like symptoms ('the nose and eyes run continually') increase until the fourth day, when

> *'Little red spots like flea-bites begin to come out on*
> *the forehead and other parts of the face...these...cluster*
> *together, so as to mark the face with large red blotches...*
> *the spots spread themselves by degrees to the breast,*
> *belly, thighs, and legs...on the 9th day they quite*
> *disappear and...the face and members seem as it were*
> *to be sprinkled with bran.'*

He added that as the rash faded respiratory complications often became severe. For this, and if there is diarrhoea, he advocated bleeding 'from the arm freely, once, twice, or thrice, as the case may require'. He was an enthusiastic bleeder, and noted that many patients with smallpox died because not enough blood was drawn off!

Sydenham was the founder of clinical medicine, and his writings were the English doctor's bible for more than a hundred years.

Measles is another of those diseases that could not have been present in hunter–gatherer communities in prehistoric times (Box 33), because you need a population of about half a million to keep measles going. However, the earliest cities, such as Uruk, Mesopotamia, in 3500 BC, had no more than 50,000 people, and actual cities of half a million have existed only since the late 17th century. Even up to the year 1800 less than 2% of Europeans lived in cities of more than 100,000. But the half million need not be concentrated in one place. If there were good communication between different towns and cities, measles would have the run of a large enough population.

The original source of the virus seems to have been the animals kept by humans. The dog (domesticated about 12,000 years ago) had the disease called distemper, and cattle (kept for food for the past 11,000 years) had rinderpest. Both diseases are caused by viruses very closely related to measles, and molecular studies point to rinderpest as the culprit.

We do not know just when the disease measles became established in humans. Perhaps there were one or two abortive, dead-end outbreaks to start with. The earliest epidemic of what could possibly have been measles was the Plague of Athens (430–429 BC) which killed off a quarter of the Athenian army before it died out. The population of Athens was about 155,000.

Measles can be particularly severe if you miss out on childhood infection or vaccination and get it when you are an adult. The King of Hawaii died of it when it was brought to his country by 19th century sailing ships and the effect of age is well illustrated by the 1846 epidemic in the Faeroe Islands. These isolated islands had been free of measles for a long time, and when it was reintroduced by an infected carpenter arriving from Copenhagen nearly everyone (about 6000) became infected, with the exception of 92 people who had survived the last epidemic 60 years earlier. The mortality was highest (28%) in infants less than a year old, but was very low (0.3%) in the 1–30 year age group, rising steadily with age to reach 8–10% in those over 60.

In those days before the development of a vaccine, measles was an almost universal childhood infection. It spared no one. The English humorist

Jerome K. Jerome (1886) noted that 'Love is like the measles, we all have to go through it.' Another English writer, Douglas Jerrold (1803–1857) adds that they are both worse when they come late in life, which is certainly correct for measles. It is one of those infections that are made much more severe by malnutrition, and in parts of Africa, where it is often life-threatening, there is an ancient Arab saying that you should not count your children until the measles has passed.

Underlying facts

The virus enters the body after being inhaled in droplets, but causes no local damage, and as in most infections, you are not aware that it has happened. It then has an intriguing step by step invasion plan (see Figure 19). After reaching the local lymph nodes it enters the blood, and then invades lymphoid tissues all over the body (see Glossary). It stays there, in the heart of the immune system, for about a week, slowly multiplying, while the child remains perfectly well. Having done its business in the immune system, the virus reinvades the blood, and this time it is seeded out onto the respiratory tract and the skin. Multiplication now begins in earnest and after a few more days (9–10 days after infection) large amounts of virus appear on the mucous membranes of the conjunctiva, nose and lungs. The child develops a running nose, red eyes, feels unwell, seems to have a bad cold, and is extremely infectious. Inside the mouth and on the skin, places that are covered by several layers of cells, it takes a day or two longer for the virus to reach the surface. When this happens inside the cheek small red spots

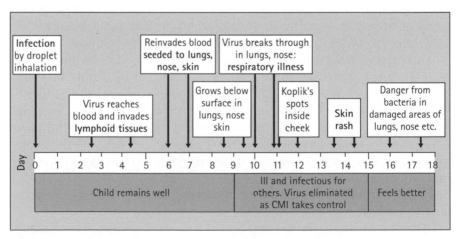

Figure 19 The step by step invasion plan of measles.

become visible (Koplik's spots) and the diagnosis can now be made for sure. Finally, 12–14 days after the virus entered the body, Sydenham's unmistakable red blotchy rash appears.

Meanwhile the immune system has not been idle. Antibodies have been formed, but it is a good CMI response that is required to clear the virus from the lungs and skin and eliminate it from the body. The virus, however, was up to no good during its week in lymphoid tissues. It caused a temporary depression of immune responses, something that was needed to give it time to complete its 7–10 day invasion plan. The effect on immunity is shown when children that normally would respond positively to skin testing with tuberculin (see Glossary) become temporarily negative on the first day or two of the measles rash. This particular fact is not irrelevant because it means that measles makes tuberculosis worse, and vice versa.

By growing in and destroying the cells lining the nasal passages and lungs, measles interferes with the local defences outlined in Chapter 2. Resident bacteria now have the opportunity to multiply in the damaged areas, spread down into normally sterile places, and cause bronchitis, pneumonia, and middle ear infections. The child then needs treatment with antibiotics. Measles still kills about a million children each year, but the WHO hopes that its energetic mass immunization campaigns will eliminate the disease from the world by the year 2010! Already, thanks to the vaccine, there are many doctors in developed countries who have never seen measles and who would have difficulty diagnosing it.

TYPHOID; A TRAIL OF ILLNESS FROM A SLIPPERY COOK

Mary Mallon was from Long Island, New York, and in 1901 she got a job as a cook with a family in New York City. Soon afterwards the family washerwoman and a visitor to the house became ill with typhoid (enteric fever). Mary then moved to another job, and a few weeks later all seven members of this family plus two of the servants went down with typhoid. More cases of typhoid cropped up in towns in Long Island in 1904, all from families where Mary had been employed as a cook. It was in 1906, when she moved to another household and six of the family developed typhoid, that the authorities went to see her and tried to dissuade her from working as a cook. She was indignant at the suggestion that she was carrying a dangerous germ.

Mary then disappeared until 1907, when there was a report that she had resurfaced as a cook in a house in Manhattan. She fled before she could be caught. The chase was now on, and eventually she was apprehended and taken for investigation, as a result of which she promised to come back for regular checks, and promised not to work again as a cook. She didn't keep either of these promises and was arrested and put in an isolation hospital on North Brother Island, off the Bronx. But Mary knew her rights, appealed to the US Supreme Court, and she was released in 1910 with another promise not to work as a cook. Then in 1914, typhoid epidemics broke out in a sanatorium and in a hospital where she had been a cook and had left in a hurry. At long last Mary was traced to a house where she was living under a false name. In the interests of public safety she was detained permanently in North Brother Island, where she died in 1938.

Mary had suffered from typhoid earlier in life, had made a full recovery, and it was in her gall bladder that the deadly bacteria had been living for so many years, reappearing intermittently in her faeces and leaving that trail of illness. In her cooking career she had been responsible for at least 200 cases of typhoid in eight different families, and had started off seven epidemics of the disease. Today's public health officers would surely have intervened with greater firmness at a much earlier stage, and the public would have been aware of the problem. Doubtless she was a superb cook.

Underlying facts

Typhoid is not a good name for the disease because typhoid just means 'typhus-like' and typhus (see Glossary) is a quite different condition. The two got mixed up so easily that typhoid came to be called *enteric fever*, which is a more accurate description of the disease. It is caused by the bacterium *Salmonella typhi*; Daniel Elmer Salmon (1850–1914) was an American veterinarian and pathologist. *Salmonella* are divided up into more than two thousand different types, but *S. typhi* is the only one that is a true, exclusively human parasite. The rest infect various animals and birds and get into our food chain in poultry, eggs, milk, cream and contaminated water. When a million or more of them are ingested they cause food poisoning (diarrhoea), which is generally over in a day or two.

However, when *S. typhi* find their way into the mouth, those that are not killed by stomach acid penetrate the gut wall. This they do silently (just as with measles in the respiratory tract), and then enter lymph nodes, where they grow in macrophages. Once they reach the blood they have access to macrophage-rich organs like the liver and spleen (see Figure 9) where further multiplication takes place. The bacteria now re-enter the blood, are seeded out along the intestinal wall and cause ulcers from which they pass into the faeces in large numbers. The great English scientist and architect,

Sir Christopher Wren, made beautiful drawings of these ulcers. The patient stays well until about two weeks after infection, and then begins to feel ill and develops a fever as bacterial products and his own cytokines are released into the blood. He suffers from constipation rather than diarrhoea. The sickness gets worse, other parts of the body may be invaded, and sometimes the ulcers bleed badly or eat through into the peritoneal cavity (see Figure 9), which is a very serious matter. Before the days of antibiotics one or two out of every ten patients died. Recovery depends mainly on a good CMI response, which stimulates the macrophages and helps them kill off the invaders, but, as is often the case, antibody matters too.

In a few out of every hundred patients the bacteria manage to stay on in the body after recovery. They survive in the gall bladder, especially in older people, or in the urinary bladder of those suffering from schistosomiasis (see Glossary). If this happens the patient, now completely well, poses a threat to others, because the bacteria, unpredictably, irregularly, and in their millions, appear either in the faeces (from the gall bladder) or in the urine (from the urinary bladder). Carriers such as Mary Mallon have been classical sources of typhoid in countries where the disease has largely been eliminated.

Typhoid used to be common in soldiers during military campaigns such as the Boer War, where hygiene was poor. Since then outbreaks have been due to contaminated ice cream, meat, and shellfish, the latter thriving in estuaries rich in sewage and filtering off the microbes that cause intestinal infections. It remains a world problem, causing 16 million cases and killing more than half a million people each year, mostly in Asia and Africa. Carriers are common. In countries with good public health and hygiene the bacteria can no longer spread via sewage to drinking water and food (see Box 27). But they are still present in other parts of the world, ready to infect if given the opportunity. This applies to tourists visiting places like Indonesia, India and Mexico, and each year a few hundred people in the UK acquire typhoid in this way. You don't necessarily have to visit these foreign lands. As recently as 1964, 507 people in Aberdeen, Scotland, developed typhoid, and the source turned out to be canned corned beef from Argentina, which had been cooled in sewage-contaminated water after canning.

The original typhoid vaccine consists of a 'soup' of killed bacteria, and people often feel ill after receiving it. The vaccine in any case gives poor protection. A new one, which seems superior, is taken by mouth and consists of living but non-virulent bacteria. Purified surface components from the virulent bacteria also give good results.

PRION DISEASES; THE MYSTERY AND THE MENACE

The hazards of cannibalism

The small aircraft taxied along the runway, turned, and began its takeoff into the breeze. The precious cargo had started on its journey, and Carlton Gajdusek found himself wondering whether his plans would work out and it would arrive safely. It was New Guinea in 1963, and the cargo consisted of refrigerated brain, on its way to Dr Gajdusek's laboratory in Washington, DC. It was the beginning of the work for which, in 1976, he would be awarded the Nobel Prize.

Journeys inside New Guinea are not easy; it is a country of spectacular us and downs, with primitive roads and many parts only accessible by light aircraft. There would be several more days before the brain arrived and his colleague, Dr Joe Gibbs, could start their critical experiment.

Arriving in the Eastern Highlands of New Guinea in 1957, Carlton Gajdusek, an American physician and anthropologist, had encountered an intriguing new disease called kuru and, together with a local physician, Vincent Zigas, he brought it to the attention of the world.

They had come across kuru in a sharply localized area inhabited by the Fore people, who still lived in barricaded villages, practised witchcraft, and indulged in ritual cannibalism. Kuru was a chronic nervous disease, previously unknown, and involved that part of the brain concerned with balance (the cerebellum). To keep steady a person with kuru would have to sit on the ground against a tree, walking being difficult even with a stick, and there was a regular shaking movement of limbs (the word kuru means shaking or trembling in the Fore language). Sufferers gradually got worse until, after 3–24 months, they died. No one recovered. The disease was especially common in women, and in some villages half of all the women had it, and as a result women were outnumbered three to one by men.

At first they thought it could be a hereditary condition, or perhaps a disease caused by eating a toxin present in a local plant. Then another scientist pointed out that under the microscope the brains from the kuru patients looked similar to the brains of animals suffering from scrapie. Scrapie is a well-known chronic nervous disease of sheep, present in Europe for 300 years, and which can be transmitted from one animal to another, but only after a very long incubation period of a year or two. Acting on this clue, Gajdusek sent refrigerated brain specimens to his laboratory in Washington, where they injected them into chimpanzees and waited.

They had to wait 2–3 years, and then the injected animals began to sicken with a disease that was just like kuru. Evidently this strange, exotic disease was caused by an infectious agent! Yet all the lab tests for known microbes were negative, so it was something new. Gajdusek and his associates reported their findings to a startled medical world in 1966. But why was the disease restricted to this remote part of the world and how did it spread from person to person?

Gajdusek was meanwhile pursuing his anthropological as well as his medical interests, focusing on child growth and development in these primitive communities. The marriage of anthropology and medicine bore fruit when work by R. Glasse made it clear that kuru was spread by cannibalism. The incubation period was an astonishing 4–20 years.

Some cannibals eat human flesh to acquire the virtues of the dead person; they eat a valiant warrior slain in battle or symbolically eat the body of a God. Others do it simply because they enjoy human flesh ('gourmet cannibalism') – it tastes of something between pork and veal. Most people would find it distasteful. We are the only mammals who don't eat our placentas, thus missing out on an iron- and protein-rich feast (the Latin word *placenta* means a flat cake). The Fore people ate their dead as a mark of respect.

Otherwise kuru did not spread between people, not to outsiders, and no new cases have occurred in the hundreds of children born to mothers with kuru. Cannibalism ceased in the 1950s and no one born since then has suffered from the disease. Kuru has now vanished from the earth. Altogether there had been a total of 3700 cases in a population of 35,000.

I mentioned that the Fore tribe practised witchcraft. People didn't just die without reason, and they attributed the kuru deaths to sorcery. One way to locate the sorcerer was to follow the direction of the flies that flew from the rotting remains of the corpse. The second commonest cause of death in the kuru villages, therefore, was reprisal murder!

Underlying facts

The infectious agent of kuru is closely similar to that of scrapie, and they are both called prions. Prions are unique because they appear to have neither DNA nor RNA, the otherwise universal materials of inheritance. Instead, a protein arranges for itself to be replicated, as outlined on page 20. Scrapie, the original prion disease, is transmissible to several other animals, including laboratory mice (Figure 20), and using them we can determine the actual amount of the infectious agent present in an organ. Nearly all our basic knowledge comes from studies in mice. Prions are amazingly

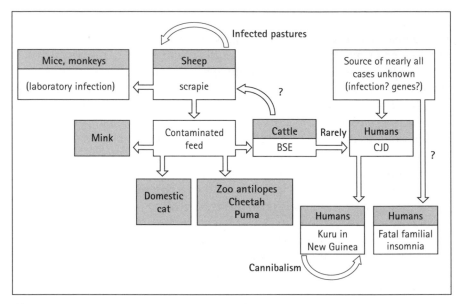

Figure 20 Prions reach out across the species. Only scrapie in sheep and kuru in humans are regularly transmitted from individual to individual, the rest are dead ends.

resistant to heat, chemical agents and irradiation. You can boil them, immerse them in formaldehyde for years, and they are still infectious. They grow in lymphoid tissues, and invade the nervous system, which is their major site of growth. The infected mouse or sheep does not become sick until prions have reached very high levels, 100,000,000 lethal doses (for mice) per gram of brain. Death comes soon after. By then the brain contains dying nerve cells and microscopic holes have formed, looking like a sponge ('spongiform'). In sheep an early sign of illness is itching, and they scrape themselves against rocks and trees to relieve this (hence scrapie). Lymphoid tissues contain only 1/10,000th as much of the infectious agent as the brain, and there is next to none in other parts of the body such as muscle, blood and milk.

One extraordinary feature of prion diseases is that the incubation period between infection and the disease is a large fraction of the life span. This means six months for mice, 2–3 years for sheep, 6–8 years for cattle, and up to 25 or more years for humans. If you were infected late in life you could die of other causes before developing the disease!

During the long incubation period the agent multiplies inexorably, and there are no signs of any immune or inflammatory response. This is to be expected if the infectious agent is a very slightly altered form of a host protein (the prion protein) which is normally present in nerve cells and immune cells, and whose function is at present unknown. As a normal body component it is not recognized as foreign.

Fifty years ago an outbreak of a scrapie-like disease in mink farms in the USA was traced to feeding the mink on material from scrapie-infected sheep, and the recent outbreak of BSE (bovine spongiform encephalopathy or mad cow disease) in English cattle had a similar origin. Transfer to various zoo animals and domestic cats has also occurred.

The equivalent disease in humans is Creutzfeldt–Jakob disease (CJD), a rare neurological disease with dementia, occurring in all continents of the world, and different from kuru. So where did kuru come from? Could it have been from a European missionary in New Guinea who had CJD, died, and was eaten by Fore people, thus starting a novel method of transmission, with changes in the disease picture?

About 10% of cases of CJD have a hereditary basis and are not acquired by infection, and recent studies on CJD have helped explain why. The gene for the prion protein has in certain families undergone a small mutation, which makes the protein more easily convertible into the abnormal form that causes the disease. Indeed it can spontaneously convert into the abnormal form, without the person ever having been infected with a prion, so that these CJD cases are based on inheritance. Here we are at the borderline of infection and heredity! As to the other 90% of cases, we still do not know where they come from. An origin from sheep has been ruled out because CJD occurs in countries like Australia where there is no scrapie.

We know now that BSE can be transmitted to people, causing a CJD-like disease ('New CJD') as a result of eating BSE-containing items such as hamburgers and sausages in the days when offal from BSE-infected cows was entering the human food chain. So far there have been 52 cases of new CJD.

CJD brains contain enormous quantities of the infectious agent, and brains and spinal cords can be dangerous to handle, especially at the stage before there are any warning signs of disease. CJD has been unwittingly transferred from person to person by the following methods:

- *Instruments used by neurosurgeons.* After use on an unrecognized CJD-infected patient the contaminated instruments (prions are not inactivated by ordinary methods of sterilization) were used on another patient and the infection transferred.

- *Injections of human growth hormone* for the treatment of children with growth failure, or of *chorionic gonadotrophic hormone* for the treatment of infertility. These two hormones are formed in the pituitary gland, which is part of the brain, and they were at one time obtained by extraction from a pool of hundreds of pituitary glands removed from dead people's brains. At that time it seemed the only thing to do, but there was an occasional brain that contained the CJD infectious agent, from someone who would later have developed CJD. This was enough to contaminate the whole batch of the hormone. Even if only very small amounts of prions were present it would be enough because the hormones are given more than once and by injection.

- *By corneal grafts and grafts of the membranes (dura) covering the brain.* Again, the source was an apparently normal person but the grafted material contained enough of the agent for it to be transferred.

Is this the end of the prion story? Prion diseases have recently reappeared in the form of fatal familial insomnia (FFI). This rare neurological disease occurs in certain families. The affected person loses the ability to sleep at 40–50 years of age, and dies a year or so later. It is a prion disease, with a special mutation in the prion protein gene, and it can be transmitted to mice (who die of it without apparently suffering from sleeplessness).

THE COMMON COLD GETS COMMONER

Cold comfort in the Arctic

The inhabitants of the islands of Spitzbergen, in the Arctic Ocean, suffer long and bitter winters. It is so far north that at this time of the year they are in almost continuous darkness for 115 days and, in the days before the aeroplane, they were surrounded by ice and cut off from the outside world. One consolation was that between December and May they were free of the snuffling, sneezing and red noses that plague other communities. City life in the English winter was described by the poet Mary Robinson (1758–1800) as follows:

> 'Pavement slippery, people sneezing,
> Lords in ermine, beggars freezing;
> Titled gluttons dainties carving,
> Genius in a garret starving.'

In May, as the temperature in Spitzbergen climbed towards freezing point, the ice began to break up, and the first ships from the outside world would arrive. They brought more than provisions and mail, because shortly afterwards a flurry of coughs and colds swept through the community. Colds could not maintain themselves for long in small isolated communities like Spitzbergen, whose over-wintering population was only 2000–3000; they had to be periodically reintroduced from outside. As argued in Box 33, this means that colds could not have existed at the time of Paleolithic man 100,000 years ago.

It may be overstating it to say that we *suffer* from common colds, and they are not severe enough to have been charted in the pages of history. But they are unpleasant, inconvenient, responsible for millions of days off work, and cost the community millions of pounds/dollars.

Underlying facts

The common cold is the name of a disease and, like hepatitis or pneumonia, it can be due to a variety of microbes. All of these are viruses, more than a hundred different ones belonging to seven different groups, with rhinoviruses (Greek, *rhinos* = nose) as the commonest. Their sheer numbers and variety tell us what a successful way of life they have chosen.

The virus is inhaled in a droplet, sticks onto cells lining the nasal cavity, and proceeds to grow in them. As the infection spreads across the sheet of cells, the early defences outlined in Chapter 2 (interferons, inflammation, phagocytes) come into action. Inflammation causes an outpouring of clear fluid, and the sneezing reflex is soon triggered off. The interferons interfere with the growth of the virus, and other cytokines in the fluid make the skin round the nose a bit sore. Polymorphs arrive at the site, attracted by a cytokine (see Glossary) called Il-8, which is released from infected cells. Already, one to two days after infection, there is plenty of virus in the fluid, and other people are infected by the sneezing, the coughing, the waving about of virus-laden handkerchiefs, as well as by hand-to-hand spread.

Cells infected by the virus are not necessarily destroyed, and nearly all the signs and symptoms of the cold seem to be due to the victim's exuberant inflammatory response. But the mucociliary defence system (see page 28, Chapter 2) is often disrupted, so that resident bacteria have the opportunity to cause trouble. If this happens the bacteria multiply, colonize the damaged areas, and in response to this more phagocytes (polymorphs) arrive on the scene. Polymorphs had already turned the nasal secretions slightly white or yellow, and now the cargo of bacteria, phagocytes and dead cells makes them thicker and cloudier.

But by this time the virus has been halted in its tracks, first because interferons (see page 42, Chapter 2) have done their work, and second because the virus begins to have difficulty finding uninfected cells. The phagocytes work hard to restrain the bacteria and clear up the debris, and if the lining cells have been destroyed they are replaced. As far as the virus is concerned it has already achieved its objective, having multiplied and spread to other people during those first few days. Immune responses have nevertheless been set in motion, and the lymphoid tissues of the tonsils often become swollen and inflamed so that the person complains of a sore throat. The antibodies formed will give resistance to this particular virus in the future.

It often takes longer to deal with the bacteria, and the unpleasant discharge from the nose may continue for a week or so. Handkerchiefs receive some of it, but most is swallowed. The sufferer notes that 'it is taking a long time to throw off this cold'.

Some of these viruses invade the cavities connected to the nose and throat, causing sinusitis or middle ear infection. Most of them grow best at the temperature inside the nose (33°C) and not at the higher temperature (37°C) down in the lungs, and they also stay in the surface layer of cells without penetrating any deeper. Those that are not so fussy (parainfluenza and adenoviruses) can descend towards the lungs and give the patient laryngitis or bronchitis.

For the forseeable future the common cold seems likely to retain its place in our species, because, as the English humorist Pam Ayres (1947–) reminds us:

> *'Medicinal discovery,*
> *It moves in mighty leaps,*
> *It leapt straight past the common cold*
> *And gave it us for keeps'*

There are no worthwhile vaccines. If you treat yourself vigorously with anti-congestants, analgesics, vitamin C, antibiotics or a whisky-lemon-honey drink, you will doubtless feel better and the cold resolves in 48 hours. If, on the other hand, you do nothing, it will probably take two days. Perhaps the scientists could make use of the idea that you, the sufferer, are responsible for most of the symptoms. They might invent a drug that worked, for instance, by stopping the action of Il-8 on your nasal passages. But over-the-counter drugs are not necessarily harmless, and in the USA in 1996 6.2% of all poisonings in children were with cough and cold remedies.

Runny noses, of course, can be due to hay fever or to other allergies, but for a proper cold you have to have the virus. It is a common belief that sitting in draughts and getting chilled causes colds, and indeed they are so-called because of this connection. Yet when volunteers were inoculated into the nose with a common cold virus and then exposed to cold by standing naked in a draughty corridor (!) their colds were no worse than in those not treated in this way. Cold weather, however, does have an effect on common colds. It has long been known that a 2–3°C fall in atmospheric temperature is followed a few days later by an increase in the number of coughs and colds in the community. This is because during the cold spell we spend a lot of the time indoors with the windows closed. Cold viruses, like the microbes causing meningitis, whooping cough or influenza, spread much more easily when we are forced to breathe other people's air.

MALARIA TRIUMPHANT

Mosquito wars

Picture the heat of southern India one debilitating day in Secunderabad, a military station, in 1897. The cooling monsoon was late this year and Dr Ronald Ross of the Indian Medical Service, back from Bangalore where he had been dealing with a cholera epidemic, had just recovered from an attack of malaria. Which was curious because his burning ambition was to get concrete proof for his theory that malaria was carried by mosquitoes. In those days it was a strange idea and many people laughed at it. Why mosquitoes? Surely you were more likely to get it from infected drinking water, or from the air? After all, the word malaria itself comes from *mal aria* = bad air.

Ross had already carried out some inconclusive experiments (unfortunately he was using the wrong sort of mosquito), and this particular day he felt disheartened. In his memoirs he recalls how, sitting in his hot, dark, little office...

> *'I did not allow the punka (fan) to be used because it blew about my dissected mosquitoes...swarms of flies... tormented me at their pleasure....The screws of my microscope were rusted with sweat from my forehead and hands, and its last remaining eyepiece was cracked!'*

But he persisted, and a month or so later, on August 16, 1897, he was studying a group of ten Anopheles mosquitoes – the right ones this time, although he was not to know it. Four to five days earlier they had been fed on a malarious patient, and each one was now being carefully dissected and examined under the microscope to see whether it carried malaria. He was down to his last two mosquitoes when, in the stomach, he saw some large pigmented objects. They were not mosquito cells and his heart beat faster. Could they be the malaria parasite? The next day he examined the last mosquito and there they were again. He later noted that 'The Angel of Fate, fortunately laid his hand upon my head.' But if these objects were the malaria parasite how did they get from the mosquito stomach into a human being? It wasn't until the following year in Calcutta, while studying bird malaria in sparrows, that he saw the parasites in the salivary gland of mosquitoes. They got there by migrating from the stomach, and the parasite was transmitted when the mosquito took a blood meal. He had noticed that a small quantity of fluid (saliva) was injected with the bite. This was the way humans were infected.

At last the problem was solved, and when his discovery was announced to the British Medical Association meeting in Edinburgh the entire audience stood and cheered (standing ovations were very rare in those days). In 1902 Ross was awarded the Nobel Prize for his pioneering work on malaria.

Much later (and not until 1948 for human malaria!), it was found that when the parasite first enters the body it makes for the liver where it establishes itself before starting its disastrous assault on red blood cells.

Underlying facts

The most important thing about malaria is that you get it from the bite of mosquitoes. Anophelene-type mosquitoes, not any old mosquitoes. Without them there is no malaria, and the best way to control the disease is by controlling the mosquito. Other key features are that it causes fever, anaemia, and sometimes a life-threatening disease, that antimalarial pills to prevent it are not at present reliable, and that the parasite can stay around in the liver for years.

The details of the complicated life cycle need not concern us. With more than 10,000 genes (humans have 80,000) its life style is bound to be complicated. There are different forms of the parasite, each adapted to the different stages in the infection of mosquitoes and humans. Each wave of infection of red blood cells causes illness and fever, and we diagnose malaria by seeing the parasite in a smear of blood under the microscope. The infection is chronic, and as the parasite invades and destroys red cells the patient suffers anaemia and debility. If the parasitized red cells clog up the blood vessels in the brain it leads to the lethal disease, cerebral malaria.

Vaccines against malaria have so far been a failure, in spite of the efforts of the world's cleverest immunologists and molecular biologists. Perhaps this is not surprising because even the natural disease does not give good immunity. Malaria is a skilled evader of host defences, and you need to suffer repeated attacks to develop resistance, which soon fades when you leave the malarious area. Both antibody and CMI are important, and repeated exposure to malaria antigens is evidently needed.

Malaria in its various forms is an ancient parasite of humans, monkeys, and of other mammals, birds and reptiles. It has long been a conqueror of people, recognized by the Ancient Egyptians, and by the Greek physician Hippocrates in 400 BC. In Ancient Rome it came from the Pontine marshes outside the city, killing children and draining the energy from the inhabitants. It killed three Emperors, stopped armies in their tracks, and possibly played a part in the downfall of the Roman Empire. In the 1930s Mussolini began to drain the marshes, and transmission of malaria finally ceased in 1948.

The disease was once common in the mosquito-ridden marshes of the Wash in south-east England. Henry VIII, Oliver Cromwell and Charles II were famous sufferers. Charles II (1630–1685) was cured of his 'ague' (malaria) by an apothecary, Robert Taylor, who gave him quinine. Quinine, from the bark of the cinchona tree in South America (Peruvian or Jesuit's bark), was introduced into Europe in 1636. The royal physicians had refused to prescribe it because of its association with Jesuits. Taylor was knighted for his actions, however, and was protected by the King from prosecution by the Royal College of Physicians as an unqualified practitioner of medicine. The disease continued in England until the last anophelene mosquitoes were eliminated in 1919.

The war against mosquitoes, which is also a war against yellow fever, dengue and filariasis (see Glossary), has been waged for a hundred years but is no nearer a conclusion. Dichlorodiphenyltricholoroethane (DDT), originally synthesized in 1874, was rediscovered in 1940 by Paul Miller, who was trying to find a chemical to control the clothes moth. In 1945 DDT was successfully tried out for the control of malaria, first along the Tennessee River, USA, and at the peak of its usage the USA were manufacturing nearly half a million tons each year. Millions of lives were saved and Miller received the Nobel Prize for his work. Mosquitoes have now become resistant to chemical sprays and the malaria parasites have become resistant to chloroquine and other drugs. About one in three people in the world are infected with malaria, suffering chronic illness and debility, and each year about two million people die of it.

LEGIONNAIRES' DISEASE; A FRESH-WATER BACTERIUM LEAPS AT THE OPPORTUNITY

The *Legionella* bacteria causing this disease live normally in patches of fresh water, in the company of amoebae and algae. The *Legionella* use foodstuffs produced by the algae, and, to survive, they have had to learn how to avoid being taken up (phagocytosed) and killed by the amoebae. They have learnt the lesson so well that they have managed to become parasites of the amoebae. This microbial trio sometimes colonizes the water in air-conditioning or water-cooling systems. They multiply and easily become airborne, suspended in small droplets of water. When people breathe them in they go down to the terminal divisions of the lung, the alveoli, where they are engulfed by local phagocytes. But the *Legionella*'s skill in coping with free-living amoebae now stands them in good stead. Rather than being killed off in the phagocyte, they multiply in it. The patient, especially the older patient, may end up with pneumonia, which fortunately can be treated with antibiotics.

The original (1976) outbreak of Legionnaires' disease was among ex-servicemen (hence 'Legionnaires') attending a meeting and staying in a certain hotel in Philadelphia, USA. Other outbreaks have been in Spanish hotels, outside the BBC buildings in London, and earlier episodes date back to the 1960s. But the infection does not spread from one person to another. Only those unlucky enough to have been in or near the particular building and inhale the original infected droplets get the disease. For this reason, although a few hundred have died, it could never, in its present form, become a common or widespread disease. The *Legionella* bacteria can be contrasted with those causing cholera (see Box 27). The latter originally were free-living inhabitants of fresh water, like *Legionella*, and occasionally infected humans. Then they mastered the art of person-to-person spread, which gave them the potential for explosive spread in crowded human communities.

I selected this disease because of its biological interest, and because it reminds us what step is needed if a microbe (*Legionella*) that is an unusual cause of a serious disease is to become one that causes a more common and widely distributed disease. This is dealt with at greater length in Chapter 10.

Part 5

WHAT THE FUTURE HOLDS

*'To complain of the age we live in, to murmur at the
present possessors of power, to lament the past, to
conceive extravagant hopes of the future, are the common
dispositions of the greatest part of mankind'*
Edmund Burke (1729–1797)

Chapter 10

THE THREAT OF NEW DISEASES

Earlier in the book I described our body's defences against parasites and the ways microbes get round these defences. Then, to illustrate the ancient conflict between microbe and host, I gave a brief account of seven human infections. In this final part I want to consider the future. Where would new infectious and possibly catastrophic diseases come from? Which of the old ones are a threat? What are our strategies for dealing with them, new or old?

I will begin with two infectious disease stories. Each is interesting in its own way, but neither of these infections, in their present form, could be serious threats to mankind.

Mousetraps save lives in Bolivia

In 1962 the small town of San Joachim, north-eastern Bolivia, was in a turmoil, afflicted by an outbreak of a severe haemorrhagic disease. It started with fever, muscle pains, a rash, and then widespread leakage of plasma (see Glossary) from small blood vessels, haemorrhage, and shock. One in five of those with the disease were dying. They were accustomed to tropical fevers, but this was an epidemic and it was different because blood-sucking insects or ticks could not be incriminated. Then the scientists had the idea that mice might have something to do with it, and they arranged for hundreds of mousetraps to be airlifted to the town. Like good investigators they set the traps first in one half of the town only, and it was soon clear that trapping mice dramatically reduced the disease. The outbreak came to an end.

A virus was finally run to earth, one that caused a harmless lifelong infection in a local species of bush mouse, and it was a member of the arenavirus family (see below). The sudden outbreak in humans seems to have arisen in the following way (see Figure 21). Because malaria was so common in the San Joachim area, extensive DDT spraying had been carried out to control mosquitoes. The geckos (small lizards that eat insects) accumulated the DDT in their bodies and as a result the town cats, that preyed on the geckos, began to die of DDT poisoning. This in turn allowed the bush mice to invade human dwellings, and people were infected by the virus excreted in mouse urine and faeces.

Luckily there was no spread of the infection directly from person to person, and without the mice in the town the disease disappeared. They called it Bolivian Haemorrhagic Fever. Lassa fever and Argentinian Haemorrhagic Fever are similar life-threatening diseases caused by arenaviruses, all carried by local species of rodents. In other parts of the world, without those rodents, and as long as they are unable to spread directly from person to person, these infections cannot maintain themselves.

But what a lesson in ecology! You interfere with Nature and the chain of cause and effect is totally unexpected.

A death-dealing military laboratory

Early in 1980 there were reports of an epidemic of anthrax (see Glossary) in Sverdlovsk, a city of 1.2 million situated 1400 km east of Moscow. The death toll was 164. The official story was that the outbreak was due to eating the meat of animals infected with anthrax, or contact with such animals. Anthrax had indeed been occurring in sheep and cattle in the area, but only sporadically and not in humans. The infected people became very ill with fever, cough, headache, chest pain and pneumonia. A voluntary vaccination programme was begun: buildings and trees were washed by local fire brigades, bodies of the dead were placed in coffins with chlorinated lime in special areas of a city cemetery and stray dogs were shot.

Foreign observers were not allowed into the city, but in 1991 Boris Yeltsin directed his officials to investigate the origin of the epidemic, and eventually in 1992 a group of scientists from the USA and elsewhere was given permission to visit Sverdlovsk.

The KGB had by then confiscated all hospital and public health records of the epidemic, but from pathologists' notes on postmortems it was clear that the fatal cases had been infected by inhaling the bacteria. What could

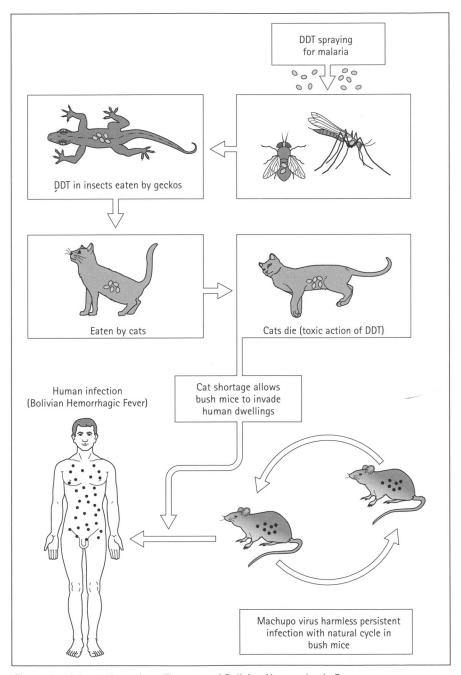

Figure 21 A lesson in ecology. The story of Bolivian Haemorrhagic Fever.

have been the source? The visiting team did a great deal of detective work, looked at grave markings in cemeteries, studied maps of the city, and found out exactly where the victims lived and worked.

The conclusions were clear, and were published in the prestigious journal *Science* in 1994. The fatal cases all lived or worked in a narrow zone extending 4 km downwind from a military microbiology laboratory. The date of onset of the epidemic, together with records of wind directions and speed, pinpointed the infections as having occurred on Monday, April 2, 1979. The first cases were seen on April 4.

There is no information as to what was going on in the laboratory or how the bacteria came to be released into the air. Anthrax can enter the body through the skin or the intestine, but the most deadly form of the disease is when it is inhaled. It has been calculated that a person needs to inhale at least 10,000 anthrax spores for the infection to be regularly fatal, although as few as ten may suffice. The total amount of anthrax escaping from the laboratory would have been less than a gram of spores, perhaps only a few thousandths of a gram, but would have contained millions of bacteria.

Anthrax is still top of the list as an agent of germ warfare, but its use depends on wind movements, and the spores stay around for 60 years. In the last analysis there are few or no moral rules in war (although it is worth having rules if everyone obeys them), and during WW2 each side had the germ warfare possibility in mind. Churchill proposed having a reserve of anthrax cluster bombs, just in case, each consisting of a hundred 4 lb units. ('Be the cad rather than the gentleman' he said.) The bombs would scatter the spores widely, and 2700 heavy bombers could seed disease and death into six major German cities. Tests in 1942 with a 25 lb bomb on the Island of Gruinard off the coast of west Scotland killed all the sheep and made the Island uninhabitable for more than 50 years.

We now have the capacity to devise things worse than anthrax, lethal infectious agents that would spread rapidly from person to person in unvaccinated (enemy) populations. Chemical warfare, however, has so many advantages that would seem a preferable option. Indeed a chemical agent that caused unconsciousness for 24–48 hours when inhaled, with no unpleasant after-effects and no damage to the environment, might be better than the guns and bombs of conventional warfare!

We can ask why anthrax bacteria release that toxin. What good does it do them as parasites to kill off so many of the infected hosts? It could be that the bacteria, basically 'saprophytic', living in soil, do not need the vertebrate host, whose death is from their point of view accidental. Or perhaps it is worth while because the dead host, with its purifying tissues, is a perfect culture medium, giving a rich harvest of spores for contaminating the environment and thus spreading the infection.

OLD DISEASES REMAIN AS A THREAT

In Part 4 we saw how the great advances in public health and hygiene, which began in the 19th century, virtually eliminated many infections from the developed countries of Europe, North America and Australasia. Cholera and typhoid retreated when something was done about sewage, water supplies and personal hygiene. Typhus, the plague and malaria became historical curiosities when lice, rats and mosquitoes ceased to be our regular companions. Many childhood infections were vaccinated out of existence.

All this has taken place in 'clean' areas of the world, where there is good sewage disposal, clean water supplies, good housing, doctors and hospitals. The old infections still flourish in other less privileged parts of the world, and when we visit them we need to protect ourselves with vaccines or medicines. They are still out there, waiting in the wings, ready to come back if there is a breakdown in the public services that go with developed societies. Cholera, typhoid, the plague, malaria and unpleasant worm infections could return to London under the right circumstances, and diseases like whooping cough, diphtheria and poliomyelitis would make a comeback if there was a serious breakdown in vaccination services. This is what happens following natural disasters such as famines, floods, wars and earthquakes. After the breakup of the USSR routine vaccination was neglected and diphtheria reappeared as a public health problem.

Rabies, for instance, could return to places where it has been eliminated. Countries like England would soon cease to be rabies-free if we relaxed our control of this disease, which is by quarantine, vaccination and reduction of infection in wildlife. Rabies was a fact of life in England two hundred years ago. It is easier to keep rabies out of islands, and it was eradicated from Great Britain by 1902. Unfortunately an illegally landed dog reintroduced it in 1918 and it was not until 1922, after 328 cases of rabies in animals, that it was once more eradicated.

Typhus tends to return when the human body louse returns, for instance in wars, and this was the case in Naples at the end of WW2. When US armed forces entered Naples they found themselves in the middle of a typhus epidemic. It was winter, and there was a shortage of clothes, soap and water, so that *body lice* were common. The epidemic was terminated by a vigorous programme of delousing. The newly discovered magic substance DDT was dusted as a powder beneath the underclothes of all the inhabitants. Typhus spreads from person to person exclusively by lice, and without the lice the disease cannot maintain itself.

Malaria, and other diseases carried by mosquitoes, could return to their old haunts if given the opportunity. Malaria was once endemic in England, as mentioned on pages 209–211, Chapter 9, and Italy was not declared malaria free until the 1920s. But in southern Italy the anophelene mosquitoes are still there, ready to start the deadly malaria cycle if the parasite gets a foothold.

It was the Europeans who brought malaria (plus yellow fever) to the Americas at the time of the slave trade. As recently as the 1930s and 1940s there were about four million malaria cases a year in the southern States of the USA. The global eradication programme of the 1950s and 1960s failed, and malaria remains one of the most intractable of the old diseases. We now face insecticide-resistant mosquitoes and drug-resistant malaria parasites.

Some of the old infections are forever restricted to particular parts of the world because they depend on wildlife or biting insects that are present only in those parts of the world. As illustrated in the example of Bolivian Haemorrhagic Fever at the beginning if this chapter, you get infected only by contact with these animals or insects, and there is no spread directly from one person to another. The tsetse flies that carry trypanosomiasis and the snails that are necessary for schistosomiasis are not present and probably could not survive outside Africa, and therefore these infections are restricted to Africa. The visiting tourist, missionary or soldier is vulnerable.

We may feel relieved at the thought of this global segregation of infectious diseases, but we need to remind ourselves that even in the 'clean' countries a few of the old diseases are holding their ground, even expanding. This includes tuberculosis (see pages 152, 168–172), sexually transmitted diseases such as HIV, gonorrhoea, genital warts and, of course, the ubiquitous common cold-type infections spread by droplets.

WHAT DOES IT TAKE TO ERADICATE A MICROBE, ONCE AND FOR ALL?

A microbe, like any life form, can be eliminated permanently, wiped off the face of the earth, made extinct. No one anywhere in the world is infected, and as long as the microbe does not survive for long in the environment, it has ceased to exist. Although this has doubtless happened once or twice in human history (e.g. the Sweating Sickness episode, page 16), it was not until recently that it took place as a result of a deliberate effort by human beings. The amazing story of smallpox eradication is outlined in Chapter 7.

The requirements are that it is an exclusively human infection, it does not stay around in the body, there is a cheap and effective vaccine and there are the resources and organization to carry out the programme.

Are there any other candidates for global eradication? Infections that fulfil the requirements include poliomyelitis and measles. Measles has already been more or less eliminated from North America by energetic vaccination, and any cases introduced from other countries are identified and their contacts vaccinated, as used to be done with smallpox. Poliomyelitis appears to have been banished from North and South America, with no reported cases for six years, and the Western Pacific region, including China, has been free for two years. The virus is still active in Africa and Southeast Asia. Of course, these infections could always return, but the WHO hopes to have eradicated polioviruses worldwide by the end of the year 2000, although in India it will take a Herculean effort. Measles is next on the list. Other infections that could be eliminated and are worth eliminating include whooping cough, diphtheria, hepatitis A, and bacterial dysentery, although in the latter case a good vaccine is still needed.

Needless to say, the benefits of eradication in relation to the costs are tremendous. The WHO estimates that US $20 billion have been saved since the eradication of smallpox in 1977. These are the purely financial savings from no longer having to provide vaccination and medical care, quite apart from the thousands of deaths and millions of disfiguring diseases avoided each year.

WHERE WOULD NEW DISEASES COME FROM?

Most species of animals and plants become vulnerable to infectious diseases when they are crowded together in large numbers. This is so for intensively reared chickens, for plagues of rodents, fish in fish farms, and 'monocultures' of food-producing plants. You can see how a microbe that spreads easily could wreak havoc under these circumstances. Indeed, it is self-evident that microbes have greater opportunities for spread in crowded human populations, and since the birth of towns and cities plague and pestilence have played a large part in human history. We do not know what most of them were. From contemporary descriptions diagnosis is almost impossible, and we can only guess at what caused the Plague of Athens (430-429 BC) or the English Sweating Sickness in the 15th to 16th century.

Today, our crowded populations are exquisitely vulnerable to respiratory infections, which spread so fast from person to person by the droplets sprayed out during coughing and sneezing. We live in a world of rapidly evolving, ruthless microbial parasites, and sooner or later something unpleasant is likely to rear its head. Not an interesting new disease that you can only catch from a rodent or biting insect in some isolated part of the world. Even if it kills, this sort of infection cannot be a threat to the rest of us unless it has learnt the trick of spreading directly from person to person. HIV (AIDS) came to us from African monkeys but it gives us no more than a foretaste of what could be in store.

The effect of crowding is not only on infections where the microbe spreads directly from person to person by droplets. It is also true for infections we get from the animals that come to live with us in our cities. *Plague*, for instance, is a natural, harmless infection of wild rodents, but when black rats became regular residents in the towns and cities of northern Europe, sometime between the 5th and 12th centuries, the stage was set for epidemics of bubonic plague, as outlined in Box 24. Even more devastating outbreaks were possible when plague bacteria invaded the lungs, so that the infection could spread by droplets from person to person ('pneumonic plague').

Another thing that influenced the expansion of infectious diseases was *clothing*. As humans colonized the cooler zones of Europe and Asia clothes became a regular feature of urban life. This had an impact on the evolution of syphilis from yaws, as described in Box 36. Clothes also provide an excellent home for lice and fleas, and when they are not washed or changed body lice can flourish. When St. Thomas a Becket, the Archbishop of Canterbury, was undressed for burial after his assassination on December 29, 1170, a thriving population of disciples was revealed in his undergarments.

> 'Outermost there was a large brown mantle; next, a white surplice; underneath this, a fur coat of lamb's wool; then a woollen pelise; then another woollen pelise; below this the black cowled robe of the Benedictine order; then a shirt; and finally, next to the body, a tight-fitting suit of coarse hair-cloth covered on the outside with linen, the first of its kind seen in England. The innumerable vermin which had infested the dead prelate were stimulated to such activity by the cold, that his hair-cloth, in the words of the chronicler "boiled over with them like water in a simmering cauldron".'

Body lice, which evolved from head lice, carry epidemic typhus (see Glossary). We can go further than this and say that clothing, by providing a new environment for a new species of louse, was responsible for the actual evolution of the body louse from its ancestor, the head louse.

Where would a new and virulent infection come from?
There are four possibilities:

1. A change in an old human microbe. Very possible.

2. Something nasty either from wildlife (mammal, bird, biting insect) or from the environment (as in the case of Legionnaires' disease and cholera).

3. Something produced by scientists 'accidentally' or for military purposes. Conceivable, but improbable.

4. Something from outer space. An impossible fantasy, in my opinion.

Let us look more closely at the first three possibilities.

1. A change in an old microbe

A new disease could be caused by a change in an old microbe. Our oldest, original collection of microbes came down with us through the ages as we evolved from the higher apes. True humans appeared about two million years ago, and the only infections that could have survived in the early nomadic hunter–gatherer communities were the small group that persisted in the body (Box 33), those that came from biting insects and those that persisted in the environment because they had spores or cysts. But human infections have arisen since those days, and I use the word old for anything that has been around for more than a hundred years.

Influenza is a likely source of a new disease because of the unique method by which a totally new type of virus is produced (see Box 15). The big change takes place quite suddenly when a bird and a human strain get together, and the new one is so different from the old ones that no one has any immunity. It will spread across the world at the speed of passenger aircraft, and if we are unlucky it could be a killer. It might, for instance, invade the lung to such an extent that fluid and cells pour into the airways and breathing is impossible. Or it could invade the heart or the brain and do a lethal amount of damage in these organs. Luckily the new strain that came in 1997 from chickens in the bird markets of Hong Kong, killing six of the 18 people infected, failed to spread from person to person. You could only catch it from chickens.

2. Something nasty from wildlife

This is the usual source of new human infections. They arise from infections already present in animals or biting insects (Figure 22).

It happens by stages. *The first stage is when the microbe jumps across from the wildlife species and infects humans, but cannot then spread directly to other humans.* The infection is therefore restricted to the places where people encounter the infected animal or insect. One interesting example is *monkeypox.* This is a virus infection of monkeys in Central and West Africa, and it was a worry during the Smallpox Eradication Programme (see Chapter 7). Africans who came into close contact with infected monkeys because they killed and ate them, became infected and suffered a small-pox-like illness. Only 400 people are known to have been infected, but the worrying thing was that it occasionally spread directly from person to person. Might it take off as a self-sustaining human infection, independent of its monkey origins? Fortunately it is transmitted very inefficiently compared with smallpox, and the longest chain of human infection ever observed was through four person to person transfers. After that it came to a dead end. But it could change!

Perhaps *plague* is in the same category. Although humans are generally infected by the bite of an infected rat flea (bubonic plague), it can also be spread directly between people by droplets (pneumonic plague). But it cannot keep going and maintain itself for long in the pneumonic form. Presumably there are inefficiencies in this method of spread, and the line of person to person infection eventually peters out.

It turns out that a great variety of human infections, some of them highly virulent, have got no further than this first stage. I'll give four examples.

Arenaviruses

A sick patient arrives at the local hospital in West Africa and dies shortly afterwards. This is not an unusual event. But when the doctor does a post-mortem, wearing gloves, and cuts through the chest to examine the heart he gets a scratch from the cut surface of a rib. A few days later he feels ill and the next week he is dead. During his illness his throat is very sore,

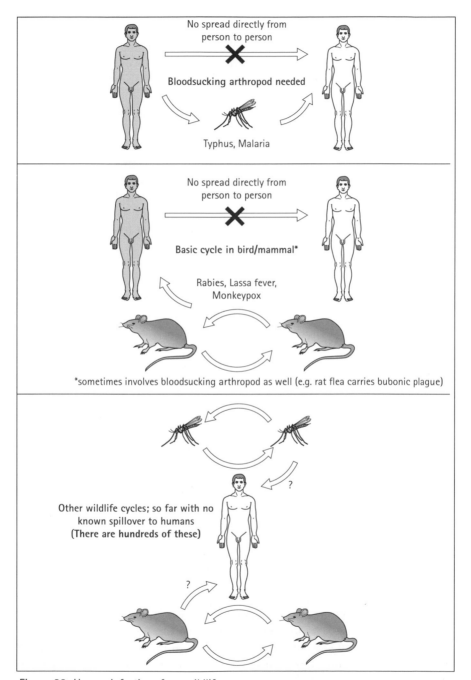

Figure 22 Human infections from wildlife.

and a nursing sister gently wipes it with a wet swab. Unfortunately she has gathered some roses from her garden that morning and has a small scratch on one of her fingers. Within a week she, too, is dead. This disease, *Lassa fever*, hit the headlines in 1970, and it seemed like a major threat to human beings.

Lassa fever is caused by one of a group of 10–12 different viruses (arenaviruses), each of which infects a certain species of rodent (see page 160, Chapter 8). Another of the arenaviruses causes the disease Bolivian Haemorrhagic Fever, which is described at the beginning of this chapter. These viruses stay in the rodent for life and generally do no harm. They are excreted in urine, and humans are infected after coming into contact with infected rodents.

The culprit in Lassa fever is an innocent-looking local species of rat, which takes up residence in native houses, excreting its virus in urine so that people get infected.

But Lassa fever *fails to spread directly* from person to person by droplets or by mere body contact. To get it from infected people you need to be inoculated through a scratch or cut with their blood or tissues, like the doctors and nurses described above. So far a dozen people, sick with Lassa fever, have been carried from West Africa to Europe on ordinary commercial airline flights in open cabins, without infecting anyone else.

We now know that infection with this virus is quite common in certain parts of West Africa, and generally causes no more than a feverish illness. People are infected by inhaling or eating a trace of virus that originated from rat urine. The doctors and nurses suffered lethal diseases because they had inadvertently inoculated themselves with the much larger amounts of the virus present in the blood or tissues of sick patients.

Ebola virus

This is another exotic virus that has caused dramatic outbreaks in southern Sudan and in Zaire. In the first two outbreaks in 1976, there were 466 cases and 311 of them died! No one knows where this virus comes from, what animal or biting insect, but outbreaks begin when an infected person turns up at hospital with a fever. He or she is given an injection of, say, penicillin, and in such parts of the world the same syringe or needle is often used for another patient without being properly sterilized. The infection spreads. It can spread through the hospital until a large proportion of the doctors and nurses are laid low, most of them dying, and in one case the army closed the hospital to contain the outbreak. These are dramatic events and have stimulated books and a Dustin Hoffman movie called *Outbreak*.

Ebola virus is still out there, keeping going in its mysterious wildlife cycle, and in 1996 another 20 human cases, with 13 deaths, were reported from Gabon, Africa. Many of these had had direct contact with the blood of dead monkeys. Are the monkeys the wildlife cycle, or did they get it from somewhere else?

Fortunately Ebola virus, like the virus of Lassa fever, did not spread to other people except by direct contact with infected blood and tissues. There was no spread by the potentially disastrous droplet method. The total number of deaths was in the hundreds, but in their present form such viruses are no threat to mankind. Locally terrifying, medically fascinating, but restricted to particular areas of the world.

There are more Ebola-like viruses out there in the wild. In 1967 a closely related virus suddenly appeared in a laboratory in Marburg, Germany. It originated in monkeys imported from Africa, and a few laboratory workers were infected and died. No one discovered exactly where in Africa the virus had come from. In 1989 yet another virus of the same type was inadvertently introduced into a laboratory in Reston, Virginia, USA. It came from crab-eating macaque monkeys that had been imported from the Philippines, and it spread among the monkeys by droplet infection and killed many of them. A few lab workers were infected but luckily it caused no illness and did not spread from person to person.

Hantaan virus

During the war in Korea (1950–1953), thousands of United Nations troops suffered from a condition called Korean Haemorrhagic Fever. It was subsequently (1978) shown to be caused by a virus picked up from local rodents, and it invaded the human kidney to give a severe disease, with 5–10% mortality. But there was no spread from person to person. The virus was named Hantaan virus, the name of a local river. Then, a few years ago, a very similar virus was found to be causing a lethal lung disease in south-western States of the USA. Like the Korean strain, it came from local rodents (deermice), but this one invaded small blood vessels in the lungs and caused an outpouring of fluid into the lungs that so far has killed 26 people. Once again, there was no spread from person to person.

The list of unpleasant infections from wildlife could go on. The recent measles-like virus that in 1994 suddenly emerged and killed 14 horses in Queensland, Australia, comes into this category. It killed one human in close contact with the diseased horses, but once again did not spread to other people. It looks as if the reservoir of wildlife infection could be in fruit bats.

Viruses from blood-sucking insects and ticks

As a final example of unpleasant possibilities from wildlife there are about 500 different viruses, mostly in the tropics or subtropics, that infect blood-sucking insects (midges, sandflies, mosquitoes) or ticks. The viruses grow in the insect or tick but they do no harm there, and this is true also of other types of microbes such as malaria or typhus. It makes sense, because if the insect or tick was damaged it would not be able to transmit the infection.

Twenty or thirty of these viruses infect domestic animals, and about 40 cause disease in humans, famous examples being yellow fever and dengue, but here, too, the infection does not spread directly from one person to another. You don't get it unless you are unlucky enough to be bitten by an infected mosquito of the right type, in the right part of the world. For the rest of these viruses, mostly found in mosquitoes, the natural wildlife cycle is unknown. If they infect humans it is on a small, unrecognized scale, and obviously the infection does not spread directly between people.

Viruses of this type are different from the three wildlife examples mentioned above (Ebola, Hantaan, and arenaviruses) because many of them are regularly being injected into humans by blood suckers, especially mosquitoes. These viruses grow in the mosquito's salivary gland, and during feeding little puffs of saliva are injected under the skin to stop the blood clotting. Only the female bites and she needs the blood if she is to lay fertile eggs. Not all species of mosquitoes find humans attractive, and the likelihood of being injected with a virus depends on how many of the mosquitoes carry it. But each infected bite gives a wildlife virus the opportunity to show what it can do in a human being. People in mosquito-ridden countries endure a surprising number of bites, in villages in coastal Tanzania, for instance, as many as 800 bites per person per day. This may not be typical, but allowing for seasonal variations, it could mean 10–100,000 bites a year!

Other microbes spread by blood suckers include malaria, sleeping sickness, Lyme disease (see Glossary), bubonic plague, typhus, and the parasitic worms responsible for elephantiasis (filariasis, see Glossary).

The second and crucial stage is reached if the infecting microbe now learns how to be transmitted directly from person to person. In theory any of the microbes that have reached the first stage could take this extra step. It means a commitment to the human species, not such a bad thing from the parasite's point of view when you remember that humans are progressively taking over the earth and most wildlife species are doomed to extinction. But clearly it is not an easy step, and microbes cannot take it just because it is theoretically possible. There are one or two examples. The probable origin of measles from a similar type of virus in cattle (rinderpest) has been referred to in Chapter 9, the origin of HIV from African monkeys and the origin of our HTLV1 from the pigmy chimpanzee, on pages 179–180, Chapter 8.

Once this stage has been reached the impact on human beings depends first, of course, on the virulence (the severity of disease), and second on the method of spread.

Cholera is caused by a microbe that arose from bacteria present in the natural environment (water), and then developed the capacity to spread directly from person to person. Legionnaires' disease, on the other hand, (see page 212, Chapter 9) arises from the environment but has failed to take that next step and is not transmitted from person to person.

A microbe that spreads by the sexual route makes its way at a moderate speed through the community, and is controllable by mechanical barriers (condoms). Spread by the faecal–oral route can be dealt with by attention to public hygiene (sewage disposal, water supplies, etc.) and personal hygiene.

A microbe that uses the droplet route, however, travels rapidly across the world, and with great efficiency. Far superior to the sexual route. By means of droplets you can infect a dozen people during an innocent hour in a crowded room, a feat far beyond the capacity of the most energetic lover. We constantly and unavoidably inhale each other's respiratory discharges. Masks are inefficient, and properly filtered air, although it can be provided in special areas like schoolrooms, laboratories or hospitals, is too impracticable and expensive for all public spaces. It is exceedingly difficult to control this type of infection unless a vaccine is available, or it is susceptible to antimicrobial drugs. Antimicrobial drugs are available for most bacteria but there are very few for viruses.

An Andromeda strain?

The 1918–1919 influenza pandemic killed 20 million people, some say nearer 100 million, and by the end of the century 10–20 million will have died from AIDS. Yet in spite of the great suffering caused, these infections have involved less than 1% of the world's population, and the effect on our species has not been catastrophic. Could a much more devastating infection arise, and disrupt life on the planet by killing or seriously incapacitating a third or a half of the world's population? Sadly, the answer is yes. Microbes evolve fast, and crowded humanity is highly vulnerable. Vulnerable also and only too easily to mediaeval fear and panic. It can be argued that the threat of infectious disease is far greater than that from cancer, heart disease, accident, starvation or war. There is no 'doomsday killer bug' on the horizon, but it is worth considering the possibilities.

An Andromeda strain (from the 1965 novel *The Andromeda Strain* by Michael Crichton) is a hypothetical type of microbe that causes massive destruction of human life. For the reasons given above such a strain, if ever it arose, would probably be a virus that was transmitted directly from person to person by droplet infection. As with myxomatosis (see Box 2), it could do great damage before finally settling down to a state of 'balanced pathogenicity' in our species. The origin could be from an old human infection, from wildlife or from the environment. Imagine the appalling consequences if HIV underwent a mutation that enabled it to spread by droplets.

3. Something nasty from the laboratory?

Germ warfare is inherently less attractive to unscrupulous leaders than chemical warfare. Germs take longer to kill or immobilize people, and there is always the possibility that a man-made, multiplying, transmissible infection could threaten the user as well as the enemy. Some of the old microbes are unpleasant. In 1979 there was a leak of anthrax bacteria from a military microbiology facility in Sverdlovsk, Russia, as described at the beginning of this chapter.

Smallpox has been eliminated as a human disease (pages 153–156, Chapter 7) but the virus itself still exists in two officially recognized laboratories in the USA and Siberia. The worry is that it may exist also, unofficially, in laboratories elsewhere in the world, and could be used as a weapon by terrorists. The world's population, now largely unvaccinated, would be disastrously susceptible.

The image of the mad scientist is a powerful one. Could a microbiological Dr Frankenstein manufacture an Andromeda strain? Modern molecular engineering has certainly brought this into the realm of possibility, but it would need more than a single mad scientist. There would have to be sophisticated, expensive laboratories and dozens of technicians. It seems unlikely, but secret ('classified') laboratories, exempt from public control, especially in countries with military dictatorships, would be danger areas.

Chapter 11

OUR ANSWERS TO INFECTIOUS DISEASES

'Outside their laboratories the physicians and chemists are soldiers without arms on the field of battle'

from *Some Reflections on Science in France Pt 1,*
Louis Pasteur (1822–1895).

Human ingenuity will always come up with answers to infectious diseases. Answers that may not completely eliminate infections from the community or even from the individual, but answers that will greatly reduce their impact. Although recently bacteria have emerged that resist everything in the antibiotic armoury this is likely to be a temporary phenomenon. So many scientists are at work on the problem, probing every weakness in the chemical life of microbes, that new drugs will surely come. Let us hope these will not have too many side-effects, and that they will be used more sparingly than has been the custom. Also, in the coming years the fruits of the modern science of immunology will at last be harvested, giving us new vaccines with unprecedented solutions to infectious diseases. The frightening question has to do with time. If a catastrophic infection suddenly appeared on the scene would our laboratories respond quickly enough to prevent massive destruction of life?

But there are other human interventions beside vaccines and antimicrobial drugs. The latter are so powerful and effective that it is easy to forget the impact of the other, often simpler, measures.

HYGIENE

The hygienic answers to sexually transmitted and faecal–oral diseases, and the rather less effective ones to droplet infections, were referred to in the last chapter.

AIDS seems to have established itself in the human species, but in spite of 20 years of intensive research we still need new drugs (16 are now licensed in the USA) and a vaccine seems as far away as ever (27 different ones are being tried out just now). Yet we do have the means (condoms) that are known to prevent infection, as well as the drugs that stop mothers giving it to their children. In other words we *already have* the solution to the spread of HIV and AIDS; the problem is with implementation.

In developed countries we accept without thinking the incalculable benefits of clean water supplies, efficient sewage disposal, and food hygiene (see Box 37). The clean water gives benefit by its effect on *washing* as well as on drinking. We have been brought up to wash our hands after defaecation, but the virtues of washing apply also to a disease like *trachoma*. This blinding disease is caused by certain bacteria (chlamydia) present in eye discharges, and it is spread by fingers, flies and towels. Repeated infection is necessary, and this is likely to occur when people have too little water to wash their faces and hands each day. In parts of Mexico the disease was greatly reduced merely by supplying piped water to villages.

Box 37   We are the lucky ones

Most of the world's suffering from infectious and parasitic diseases is due to poverty. There is a great divide between the developed nations of western Europe, North America and Australasia and the rest of the world. You can illustrate this in various ways. The world's top three billionaires have assets greater than the combined GNP of all the least developed countries and their 600 million people! In these countries three out of four people die before the age of 50. Only some of these premature deaths are due to infectious disease, but vaccines, clean water and sewage treatment would cost very little compared with the amount of money spent on armaments. The divide is there, even with something as basic as spectacles for reading, working, learning, living. About 20 million people in sub-Saharan Africa ought to have spectacles, which need only cost US$2–3 a pair. And there is only one ophthalmologist for every three-quarters of a million people.

Controlling flies also makes a big impact but it has to be kept up. Worldwide about 150 million children are actively infected with trachoma, and six million people are blinded by it. The benefits of washing are well illustrated by the summary in Box 38 of a classical chapter in the history of infectious diseases.

Washing of hands and faces is a matter of personal hygiene, but water also washes clothes, which not only removes harmful staphylococci and other microbes (see Box 21), but also helps reduce infestation by body lice and other disease-carrying parasites. Unwashed, unchanged clothes have often been the background for epidemics of typhus (see Glossary).

In 1817 the Estonian surgeon Werner Zoege von Manteuffel recommended sterilized (boiled) rubber gloves to protect the patient from infection. He was the first to do so, saying that to wear boiled rubber gloves was to have boiled hands! Dirty rooms often harbour infection, especially in hospitals. There is much to be said for simply keeping places clean. Common or garden cleaning, vacuuming, etc., is often neglected and at times can be as useful as more sophisticated methods of infection control. When Florence Nightingale arrived at a Crimean hospital in the 1850s she reduced the

---

Box 38 The unpopularity of Semmelweis, and Lister's acid strategy

A hundred and fifty years ago up to one in ten of all mothers died shortly after giving birth. The newly emptied uterus is a raw wound, vulnerable to virulent streptococcal bacteria, and there were no antibiotics. So-called *puerperal sepsis* (*childbed fever*) was an accepted hazard, a fact of life, and it features in several Victorian novels. My mother died of it in 1930.

In 1847 Ignaz Semmelweis, a Hungarian doctor at Vienna Lying-in Hospital, noticed an interesting difference between two of the hospital wards. In one ward 9.9% of all newly delivered mothers died, whereas in the other ward only 3.9% did so. In the first ward medical students studying obstetrics came in straight from the dissecting rooms, without changing their blood-splattered coats or thoroughly washing their hands. Indeed the hands 'retained their cadaveric odour' for some hours afterwards. The second ward was run by midwives who were very fussy about cleanliness. Were the medical students bringing in a disease-causing material? One of Semmelweis' friends had died from blood-poisoning after cutting his finger during dissection, and the symptoms were similar to those of the mothers. Semmelweis therefore insisted that

---

Box 38 The unpopularity of Semmelweis, and Lister's acid strategy (continued)

all the students wash their hands with a lime chloride solution before entering the ward. The result was striking. The following year the mortality in the ward had fallen to 3%, and the year after to 1.27%.

But Semmelweis' methods brought him great unpopularity. None of the other doctors made a fuss about such things, and he was obviously a trouble-maker to suggest that mothers were killed by the unclean hands of medical attendants. His contract at the hospital was not renewed, and he was forced to leave Vienna. His epoch-making book, born of long and acrimonious medical disputes, was not written until 1861 when he was in Budapest. He became depressed, and in 1865 entered a lunatic asylum. He died 12 days afterwards, having received an astonishing gift from the fickle finger of fate. During one of his last operations he had cut his finger, the wound became gangrenous and death was due to streptococcal blood-poisoning. He died from the very disease he had been trying to prevent during the whole of his professional life!

At almost the same time a physician at Glasgow Royal Infirmary, Joseph Lister, a convert to Pasteur's idea that germs cause diseases, heard about the value of carbolic acid as an antiseptic agent for sewage. On August 12, 1865, 11-year-old James Greenlees was run over by a cart and suffered a compound fracture of the left leg. Lister washed the wound with carbolic acid solution and linseed oil, set the fracture, and covered it with tin foil to stop evaporation. The acid burned the skin, but the wound healed perfectly, and the patient walked home six weeks later. Under normal circumstances he would have lost the leg and probably his life. Lister's carbolic acid made surgery safer, and it acquired respectability when he used it for lancing an abscess in Queen Victoria's armpit.

Yet now, 150 years later, even doctors and other health-care workers often neglect handwashing. Horrified by lice on a patient, they ignore the invisible but potentially harmful bacteria on their own hands. Clearly not every single contact has to be followed by handwashing. Shaking hands with a well patient is different from examining an infected wound. Perhaps for busy doctors, touching 50 or more patients a day, rubbing hands in chlorhexidine or alcoholic antiseptic gels, as practised in Germany, can be an alternative to traditional handwashing. We also know that white coats, and perhaps even the ends of stethoscopes, can harbour harmful bacteria.

dysentery, cholera and typhoid death rate from 42% to 2%, largely by organizing an effective cleaning system and a proper laundry service, plus structural repair of wards. For the first time that anyone could remember the hospital floors were scrubbed. Exquisite cleanliness is required in a sick room, she said.

Spitting is another example of bad personal hygiene. It is indulged in only by humans and a few other animals such as camels, llamas, chameleons and certain snakes. Chimpanzees soon learn how to do it. Until the turn of the century it was practised by most people and was more or less socially acceptable. But campaigns against it began in the 1880s because of the fear of tuberculosis. By 1916, 195 of 213 American cities had rules against spitting in public. This was poorly enforced, and admonitory signs included: 'Gentlemen will not, and others must not, spit on the floor.' The decline of chest conditions like chronic bronchitis and tuberculosis means that nowadays, luckily, there is less spit available for ejection, and it is a less dangerous material.

Sewage disposal is a major item in the life of towns and cities, but unseen and unappreciated. The water arriving at sewage works is contaminated not only with faeces and urine but also with countless other materials. Sometimes it is run straight into the sea after being crudely filtered and homogenized so as to remove tell-tale objects. Generally it is cleaned, harmful microbes removed or killed, and safe water finally discharged into rivers. The methods used are a triumph in microbiological engineering. Take the river Thames. During the magnificent Victorian clean-up of this grossly polluted river (Box 27) a great network of sewage pipes and pumping stations was constructed which, seen on a map, remind one of the London Underground system. Since then the quality of Thames water has steadily improved. Before the industrial revolution it had been so clean that Henry VIII's polar bears in the Tower of London were let out into the river on a chain to catch their own salmon. Today the salmon are returning.

The sewage works also produce methane gas (used to generate electricity), and immense quantities of nitrogen and phosphorus-rich sludge. At present this is dumped in the sea, but one day it will have to be recycled more efficiently. Two hundred years ago London sewage was collected as 'night soil' and used to fertilize fields.

Food hygiene means the control of microbial contamination and growth in food, mostly by refrigeration and pasteurization. In pasteurization the food material (milk, cheese, beer) is given mild heat treatment for a limited period of time (63–66°C for half an hour in the case of milk). This does not kill all microbes (does not sterilize) but it deals with the harmful ones such as the bacteria causing tuberculosis, brucellosis (see Glossary) and food-poisoning, without spoiling the taste or appearance.

You can stop infection spreading by *isolation* or *quarantine* of infected individuals, and this has been used for hundreds of years. In the battle against yellow fever and bubonic plague in sea-ports, incoming ships from infected regions were required to remain offshore and not land for several weeks. The word quarantine (Italian = forty days) refers to the original period visitors had to wait before entering the city of Florence. Nowadays isolation and quarantine are not used for commonplace infections, firstly because many of them are at their most infectious stage before they are diagnosed. Secondly, because in many cases (glandular fever, chickenpox) it is better to be infected early in life rather than later (see pages 80–83, Chapter 4).

Reducing infection from wildlife. If the disease comes from dogs, cows or foxes, you can control it by killing or cleaning up that source of disease. For instance, dogs in Europe are vaccinated against rabies, and fox rabies has been reduced in Canada by dropping from aircraft bait containing rabies vaccine. The foxes eat the bait and are vaccinated.

Outbreaks of Bolivian Haemorrhagic Fever have been terminated by attending to mice (see beginning of Chapter 10).

Many of our infections used to come from cows or their milk, and the development of tuberculosis-free herds, together with pasteurization of milk, were milestones in the control of tuberculosis.

Reducing infection from biting insects and ticks. Obviously you can tackle the infections spread by mosquitoes simply by killing them or by stopping them from biting. The control of louse-borne typhus was mentioned on page 219, and for more than a hundred years humans have waged war against mosquitoes. Despite local successes in cities and islands, the war is still on. Thousands of tons of insecticides have been sprayed and marshes have been drained, but the onslaught is interrupted by wars and money shortages. The mosquitoes keep coming.

Malaria is the biggest problem. Each year about two million people die of it (90% of them in Africa) and many more suffer chronic ill health. Because the parasite has become resistant to many antimalarial drugs, the present emphasis is on preventing the mosquitoes from biting. About three-quarters of a million UK citizens a year visit malarious countries, and hundreds of them come back home and develop malaria, generally because the drugs weren't taken properly, but also because they encountered drug-resistant strains of the parasite. They are advised also to protect themselves from bites by covering arms and legs, and using insect repellents and mosquito nets.

One very promising measure for large-scale use in malaria-ridden places is the provision of bed and door nets impregnated with a biodegradable insecticide (pyrethroid). When distributed free to villages in Ghana and Kenya, hospital admissions for severe malaria fell so dramatically that it was hailed as one of the most cost-effective public health interventions ever undertaken.

ANTIMICROBIAL DRUGS

We now come to a ridiculously brief mention of one of the greatest achievements of 20th century medicine. Antimicrobial drugs (see Box 39) include *antibiotics*, which strictly are substances produced naturally by fungi and bacteria. They kill other microbes or stop them growing, and in the microbial world have always been useful weapons in the cut-throat competition for space and food. Long before penicillin, a fungal product, was discovered and used by humans, certain free-living bacteria had developed resistance to it in the age-old war between one microbe and another. Many of the modern versions of antibiotics, however, have been chemically modified, and sulphonamides and quinolones (a large group of antibacterial agents, including ciprofloxacin) are totally man-made.

Paul Ehrlich (1854–1915) was the pioneer. He had the idea that there were bound to be chemical agents (magic bullets) that were more harmful to the parasite than to the host, and he developed the arsenic-containing drug Salvarsan for the treatment of syphilis. He was denounced by the clergy for interfering with God's punishment for sin but that method of treating syphilis, together with bismuth, mercury and fever therapy, was used until the discovery of penicillin.

What everyone would like to have is a new type of drug, not toxic, not harmful to the unborn child, which has a wide range of activity, and which poses such insuperable problems to the microbe that resistance is impossible. The sort of drug that kills germs in the way that cyanide or lethal war gases kills people. An omnicillin or wondermycin! Probably there is no such drug. Meanwhile, pharmaceutical laboratories across the world continue their search for new ones, although no new class of antibiotic has been discovered for about 20 years. The most powerful approach for the scientist is based on biochemical logic. You identify vulnerable stages in the microbe's growth cycle and then develop drugs specifically designed to interfere with these stages. We can only hope that for most infections human beings keep one step ahead of the microbes.

Box 39 The antimicrobial drugs we use

- *Antibacterial agents* generally do their job by preventing bacteria manufacturing their cell wall (penicillins), by inhibiting the synthesis of proteins (tetracyclines), or by inhibiting the synthesis of nucleic acids (DNA, RNA; e.g. sulphonamides, trimethoprim, quinolones). Some of them act against a wide spectrum of microbes (tetracyclines) and others have a more focused action (the sulphonamide-like drug dapsone for leprosy).
- *Antifungal agents* are not so numerous, because fungal cells are more like our cells than are bacteria, and it is harder to find a drug that does no harm to humans. Antifungals are often suitable for use in creams or ointments on the body surface (benzoic acid, fluconazole, miconazole), but may be too toxic to use inside the body against the invasive fungi.
- *Antiviral agents* are still few and far between, in spite of intensive research efforts. This is partly because such drugs must act where the virus is vulnerable, inside the host cell, yet without damaging it. Toxicity, damage to host cells, is therefore a common problem. The meagre list of recognized antiviral drugs includes aciclovir for herpes simplex, ganciclovir for varicella zoster (chickenpox-shingles), and retrovir and other drugs for HIV. Viruses, unfortunately, can become resistant, and we already have aciclovir-resistant strains of herpes simplex and retrovir-resistant strains of HIV.
- For *protozoa and worms* we have a variety of agents, some of them quite useful, such as chloroquine for some strains of malaria, and mebendazole for many worms. Resistant strains of malaria are becoming so widespread that additional measures must be used to protect people, as mentioned above.

The menace of drug-resistant microbes

The emergence of drug-resistant malaria, gonorrhoea, tuberculosis, leprosy or staphylococci, is a sad story for patients and physicians. The microbe is always mutating, altering its DNA, and a strain with a change that makes it resistant to a commonly used drug will tend to replace the original strain.

There is no doubt that overuse and over-prescribing of these drugs encourages the emergence of the resistant strains. The drug, in other words, is a victim of its own efficacy. It happens all over the world, especially in hospitals where so many of the patients have been given these drugs.

One of the best-known examples is *Staphylococcus aureus* that resists the penicillin-like drug methicillin, the so-called MRSA (methicillin-resistant *S. aureus*). The 'M' now stands for 'multiply' rather than just 'methicillin', because these strains resist a variety of different antibacterial drugs. The pneumococcus (see Glossary) is beginning to tread the same pathway.

Other ominous examples are resistant tuberculosis bacteria. In this disease three drugs are used in combination to give the bacteria the least possible chance of developing resistance. During treatment of an infected individual, however, any bacteria that have learnt new tricks and can grow in the presence of those drugs, will blossom out. Recently strains of tuberculosis have emerged that resist all three drugs.

HIV, with its high rate of mutation, is another example. The antiviral drug Zidovudine (retrovir) by itself has been very disappointing, and the result is much better when two other drugs are given at the same time. The patient lives longer and the disease progresses more slowly. Will there be virus strains that resist all three drugs?

Adverse drug reactions

Drugs work wonders and have transformed the treatment of many diseases. Yet there are few drugs that are completely harmless. Aspirin can cause serious bleeding, and in some people penicillin causes severe allergic (anaphylactic) reactions. A recent (1998) study gave the surprising result that adverse drug reactions accounted for more than 100,000 deaths each year in the USA. They only included drugs that were correctly prescribed and administered. It was the fourth commonest cause of death after heart disease, cancer and stroke. The exact figure is perhaps open to question, and some might argue that it is not excessive when considered in relation to the human suffering prevented and lives saved by drugs. But it serves to remind us first, that there is not a magical drug to cure every human ailment, and second that in each case the possible harm to the patient has to be balanced against the probable benefit.

VACCINES

First, what is a vaccine?

It is a material from a microbe which, when introduced into the body, stimulates an immune response to itself, and thereby prevents infection and disease due to that particular microbe. Injecting preformed antibodies (gammaglobulins) to protect against a disease such as rabies or hepatitis A is not strictly vaccination, because the person has been passively protected without having to develop his own immunity.

Vaccines are so-called because of the story of Jenner and smallpox vaccination (see pages 153–156, Chapter 7). They can be injected into skin or muscle, taken by mouth, even up the nose. A guide to the main vaccines is set out in Box 40.

What is a vaccine made of?

It can consist of the whole microbe, either killed if it is the virulent strain, or living and multiplying in the case of a harmless (avirulent) strain produced in the laboratory. Many vaccines, however, are mere fragments of the microbe, or are substances (antigens) derived from it, but they are highly effective as long as an immune response to those paticular antigens is enough to give protection. For example, when a disease is caused by a toxin (cholera or tetanus, see Chapter 8), the toxin is treated in the laboratory so as to render it non-toxic without interfering with its capacity to induce immunity. Cholera and tetanus vaccines, therefore, make you form antibody to the toxins so that disease is prevented. The pneumococcus owes its disease-producing powers to the slimy capsule surrounding it, which stops it being engulfed by phagocytes. If you extract and purify the capsule material and use it as a vaccine, the antibody formed against the capsule disarms the bacteria (see Figure 12) and pneumococcal disease is prevented.

Vaccination, which has prevented so many lethal or crippling diseases, is one of the greatest achievements of modern medicine, although its opponents are vociferous, and the public only too easily worried. Pressure groups against vaccines, like those against genetically modified foods, tend to drive public opinion, and the case for science is not always given a chance. Attention is focused on risks, both real and perceived, rather than on enormous benefits and it ends up like a dialogue of the deaf, with everyone shouting and no one listening. Public trust and confidence in vaccination is eroded. But modern science has not always been necessary. Smallpox (see Chapter 7) was eliminated by a vaccine born of logical thought, without the assistance of modern science. Many other vaccines, however, including yellow fever, measles, polio, rubella and BCG, were only developed once scientists learnt how to grow the microbe in the laboratory. The microbe was then cultivated for long periods until it had lost its virulence for humans and was a candidate for use as a vaccine. Drs Enders, Weller and Robbins were awarded the Nobel Prize in 1954 for discovering how to grow viruses

Box 40 A guide to human vaccines

Vaccine	Type[1]	Status (reliability, safety)
Measles, mumps, rubella[2], polio (oral, Sabin type), yellow fever	Live, multiplying non-virulent strains	++++
Varicella zoster[3], BCG (tuberculosis)		++
Hepatitis A, hepatitis B, polio (injected, Salk type)	Non-living non-multiplying microbes	++++
Influenza, rabies		+++
Whooping cough (pertussis)		++
Cholera, typhoid[4]		+
Tetanus, diphtheria	Inactivated bacterial toxins	++++
Pneumococcus[5], meningococcus, Haemophilus influenzae[6]	Slimy capsule of bacteria	+++

1. As a general rule, several shots of non-living vaccines have to be given to stimulate immunity, whereas living vaccines, because they grow in the body and thereby produce plenty of antigen, need only be given once.
2. Measles, mumps and rubella combined, as MMR vaccine.
3. Not yet licensed for general use in the UK.
4. A living, non-virulent strain of bacteria (Ty21a) is now available.
5. Pooled capsule material from 14 or 23 of the commonest types of pneumococcus (there are 84 types altogether).
6. H. influenzae type b, a common cause of meningitis and other severe infections in children (see Glossary).

No vaccines yet available for:-
Malaria, syphilis, gonorrhoea, trypanosomiasis, leprosy, HIV, rotavirus, nearly all of the herpesviruses, all worm infections.

in cells in test tubes, which led the way to making vaccines against polio, rubella, measles and mumps.

Who gets the vaccine?

Most vaccines are given to infants, who need to be protected early in life against diseases like measles, whooping cough, diphtheria and polio. Others are for people who risk infection because they are going to countries where the infection is common (cholera, typhoid, hepatitis A, hepatitis B, rabies), or for people who are particularly vulnerable, as in the case of influenza vaccine for the elderly and for those with heart and lung diseases. And of course there are people who should not be given live, multiplying vaccines, such as those with immune defects or pregnant women. Living vaccines can multiply unchecked in those with immune defects, and in pregnant women there is a risk of damage to the fetus.

Nearly all of us have been vaccinated against the common infectious diseases, and thus immunized. Immunization makes good medicine and is cost-effective. In my childhood I was ill with measles, mumps, diphtheria and whooping cough, and silently infected with polio and tuberculosis. Today these diseases are all but banished from developed countries, and are becoming so rare that most young physicians have had no first-hand experience of them.

Each vaccine has its own rules and its own problems

Measles, in developing countries, is most lethal during the first year of life, when the protective umbrella of maternal antibodies is waning. The problem is that this umbrella itself can prevent the growth of the live virus in the vaccine and make it ineffective. Ideally the measles vaccine should immunize infants in spite of those maternal antibodies. Again, rubella (German measles) is harmless for children and adults, but can infect and damage the fetus. Females, therefore, are the ones who need the vaccine so as to protect the future fetus. We vaccinate them to protect an as yet non-existent individual! Should you give it to schoolgirls just before they are of childbearing age, or should it be one of those given (more conveniently) in infancy, with the risk that immunity may have waned by the time they are pregnant? In the UK it is given as part of MMR, during infancy.

How do you take account of antigenic variation of influenza virus (see Box 15) and produce enough up-to-date vaccine in time for this winter's epidemic? Last year's vaccine may be no good for this year's virus. We need a new, cleaner, whooping cough vaccine, and when will it be ready? When will we have an efficient vaccine for HIV, ideally one that gives local immunity against vaginal and rectal infection? For many infectious diseases there are no vaccines (see Box 40). The scientists are trying hard but it is a slow business, and at present there are nearly 200 different vaccines in the research development stage.

There is more to vaccination than having a good vaccine

There is little doubt that improved vaccines will soon be available, but many of the difficulties are financial (the cost to poor countries), or to do with delivery (political upheavals, local wars). This is where international bodies such as the WHO and UNICEF are crucial, as was demonstrated in the Smallpox Eradication Programme (see Chapter 7), and in the Children's Vaccine Initiative.

The Children's Vaccine Initiative was a coalition of international agencies, governments and vaccine companies, set up in 1991 to foster the development and use of vaccines in children. Major successes included the elimination of polio from the Americas, and progress in eliminating measles. Also, they achieved dramatic increases in vaccination of the world's children against measles, diphtheria, whooping cough, polio and tuberculosis, from a figure of less than 5% in 1974 to 80-90% in 1994. This meant that the lives of 3.5 million children were saved each year. In a single day in India in 1999, thanks to the help of two million volunteers in 600,000 immunization centres, no less than 130 million children were vaccinated against polio.

In developed countries the antivaccination lobby presents a worrying threat to the control of infectious diseases. This is partly due to adverse and often misleading publicity about harmful effects of vaccines, and partly a general distrust and revolt against science itself, ironically among the very people whose lives have benefited most notably from advances in science. Words like 'DNA' and 'genetically engineered' (like 'nuclear' for the opponents of the world's main energy source for the 21st century) make such people suspicious or angry. The answer is to better inform and educate people about vaccines.

You can make up a league table of vaccines (Box 40)

One of the best is yellow fever vaccine, a living but harmless strain of the virus, which grows in the body and stimulates life-long immunity with no side-effects. One of the worst is the current cholera vaccine, which is no more than bacterial soup, suitably killed, but containing hundreds of different antigens, and only giving poor and short-lived protection. It would make sense if the vaccine for this disease was taken by mouth so as to generate local immunity in the intestine (IgA antibody, see page 56, Chapter 3), the place where the microbe enters the body. Instead it is injected into skin or muscle and stimulates less appropriate IgG antibodies.

The old typhoid vaccine was in the same category, but a greatly improved one is now available, taken by mouth, and consisting of living, non-virulent bacteria.

Other vaccines come in the middle of the list. The old whooping cough vaccine, for instance, another killed bacterial soup, gives worthwhile immunity but contains bacterial components that can cause unwanted side-effects. A cleaner (acellular) vaccine is available. And BCG (see Glossary), invaluable in the continuing battle against tuberculosis, is not universally effective. It doesn't protect too well against the adult form of the disease, is poorly effective in certain parts of the world and is not much use against the related disease leprosy.

Future vaccines

There are many promising new developments in vaccinology, but few of them have yet reached the stage of being licensed for general use.

Finding the right antigen
In many cases we do not know exactly which of the microbe's antigens induce the sort of immune response that will give lasting protection. This is so for tuberculosis and HIV, but scientists now have molecular tricks at their disposal, such as seeing whether or not the microbe, in order to stimulate immunity, needs the gene for a particular microbial antigen. If it does, this antigen is an essential part of the vaccine.

New adjuvants
An adjuvant is something that enhances the immune response to a vaccine, without itself being the antigen. The alum salts in the tetanus and diphtheria vaccines act in this way. An ingenious and more precise method for 'live' vaccines is to incorporate into the microbe used as a vaccine a gene that forms a substance which will stimulate immunity locally in the body. The substance could be a cytokine with a booster effect on immunity, and it would be produced wherever the vaccine happens to be growing.

Vaccine cocktails
Scientists can now assemble a number of different vaccines into a single vaccine cocktail. This is another triumph of molecular biology. Once you have discovered the antigen that gives protection against microbe x, you

take a fairly harmless live microbe that will grow in the body, and insert into its DNA the DNA (gene) for the protective antigen. When the harmless microbe infects the individual it multiplies and in the course of doing so makes large amounts of the antigen from microbe x. The person therefore becomes immune to microbe x.

The harmless microbe used to carry the gene from microbe x can be vaccinia virus, the one used in the smallpox eradication programme, or the closely related poxvirus of canaries, which is even more harmless. BCG or *Escherichia coli* can also be used. The advantage of this approach is that at least ten different genes from ten different microbes can be grafted onto the harmless microbe, and when this one multiplies ten different antigens are formed, so that you develop ten different immunities after a single shot.

Banana vaccines?

The same sort of molecular engineering can be used to introduce a gene responsible for a key microbial antigen into the DNA of a *plant*. The plant then produces large amounts of the antigen, and when you eat the plant you are vaccinated, developing mucosal (intestinal) immunity to the microbe. It has been tried out experimentally in tobacco plants for hepatitis B vaccine, and in potatoes for a vaccine against a harmful type of *E. coli*. But if the plant is smoked or cooked the vaccine's antigen would be destroyed.

A banana is a more convenient, baby-friendly alternative, the world's fourth largest crop, and foreign genes have already been inserted into banana DNA. Unfortunately this work progresses slowly because it takes one and a half years to grow a banana tree and harvest and test the crop. It has been calculated that if a single banana holds ten doses of a vaccine, all the children in the world could be vaccinated with 200 million bananas, which is only 0.2% of the total number eaten each year. Edible vaccines would be cheaper, as well as nicer, and a banana vaccine is the holy grail for these scientists.

Skin patch vaccines

This is an intriguing approach. The vaccine is soaked into a skin patch, is absorbed by local immune cells within an hour or so after applying the patch, and an immune response follows.

Can one shot do it all?

The ultimate goal of vaccinators is to invent a *supervaccine*, one that immunizes against the relevant 10–20 infectious diseases, is taken by mouth with no need for injections, only needs a single dose, and lasts forever! It would also need to maintain its potency without refrigeration (often a great problem in developing countries), and be inexpensive. This is not an impossible dream. The question is, just when will the immunologists and microbiologists be able to deliver it? A supervaccine would be an amazing gift to humanity from the scientists, who have been having a bad press in recent years. It would also be a fitting gift to the rest of the world, from those countries that have had the resources and wisdom to invest heavily in laboratory research.

DNA vaccines

Scientists were surprised to learn, a few years ago, that pure DNA could function as a vaccine. If the DNA (gene) for a microbial antigen is injected directly into a muscle of a mouse it gets into cells, and these cells, under instruction from the foreign DNA, now start to produce the antigen. As a result the mouse develops antibody and CMI to that microbial antigen, and in this way it can be immunized and protected against infection with influenza virus. However, it is not clear whether a DNA vaccine would be acceptable for human beings. Many physicians and scientists have misgivings about introducing foreign genes into the cells of human beings. Nevertheless the method has immense power and promise; currently about 40 different DNA vaccines are being developed in laboratories.

If you can't beat them, join them; genetically engineered mosquitoes

A novel idea for vaccination in countries where mosquitoes are common is to get the mosquitoes to carry out the actual vaccination. If you know the antigen that stimulates immunity and thus gives protection against a disease, you could transfer the gene for this antigen into a mosquito. Once all the mosquito's cells have the gene, the antigen will be excreted into its saliva as it bites you. This is an 'If you can't beat them, join them' approach to the mosquito problem, and could be used not only for mosquito-borne diseases like malaria but also for any other infectious disease. The problem, once the genetically engineered mosquitoes have been produced in large numbers, would be to release them into the environment and ensure that there were enough of them in relation to the regular unmanipulated mosquitoes. Who knows what might come next using this vaccination strategy?

NATURAL THERAPY

As far as infectious diseases are concerned, natural therapy means treatment with substances produced naturally by animals, plants or microbes. It is part of alternative (complementary, unconventional) medicine, whose influence has blossomed in recent years. A useful book, *The ABC of Complementary Medicine*, is to be published by the British Medical Association in Spring 2000. Patients often use natural therapy in *addition* to conventional medicine rather than as an *alternative*. One in ten people in the UK, more than one in three in France, the USA and Australia, and two out of every three in Japan, regularly visit a practitioner of complementary medicine. Included are acupuncture, chiropractice, osteopathy, homoeopathy, as well as natural (herbal) therapy. Complementary medicine comes into its own in the treatment of diseases where the cause is unknown, or when conventional doctoring has little to offer. People resort to it especially when they have chronic complaints such as arthritis or skin conditions, or when they are dissatisfied with mainstream medicine. Infectious diseases, however, are not generally included, except in the case of herbal therapy. Indeed the acupuncturist's needles, like those of the tattooist or the ear-piercer, suggest the conveyence of infection (hepatitis, HIV) rather than its cure. Also there have been examples of harmful infectious agents present in herbal products.

Antibiotics

Antibiotics, strictly speaking, are examples of natural therapy because they are produced by microbes and act against other microbes. The usual source is fungi, or certain bacteria living in soil. More than 5000 have been discovered, but they are often unsuitable because they have toxic effects, and less than one in a hundred end up being of any practical value.

It all began with Fleming, who in 1928 discovered *penicillin*, produced by the mould *Penicillium notatum*, although the discovery did not bear fruit until the work of Florey and Chain in 1941. Mice are also part of the story, because the new drug was finally used on humans after it was shown that it prevented mice dying after infection with virulent streptococcal bacteria.

Other antibiotics include *streptomycin* (1943) and *cephalosporin* (1945), the latter from a fungus recovered from near a sewage outlet in Cagliara, Sardinia. Also *rifampin* (1957) and *tetracycline* (1949), the latter being discovered by Benjamin M. Duggan, a 72-year-old fungal expert.

The natural world remains a promising source of antimicrobial substances, and pharmaceutical companies continue their search for new substances from microbes and from plants.

Quinine

This is a world-famous natural product. It has long been known that the symptoms of malaria can be treated by drinking an infusion prepared from the bark of the cinchona tree, a native of South America. The tree is called cinchona in memory of the first European on record to have been successfully treated. In 1638 the wife of the Viceroy of Peru, the Countess Cinchon, lay very ill with malaria in the Vice Regal Palace in Lima, Peru. The court physician cured her with quinquina (American Indian = bark of barks), an extract from the bark of this tree. It is interesting that another bark, from the yew tree, is the source of *taxol*, a promising new drug against cancer.

It was the Jesuits who spread the word about quinine, and on this account the great Protestant, Oliver Cromwell, was so prejudiced against it that he suffered unnecessarily. He had chronic malaria, but called quinine 'the powder of the devil' and refused treatment all his life.

The Dutch set up cinchona plantations in Java in 1854, and quinine from Java was the sovereign remedy for malaria. It was a vital ingredient in the expansion of Europeans into Africa in the 19th century, and enabled Europeans to survive in regions where they would otherwise have died. When the Japanese seized Java in 1942, the hunt began for an alternative drug, and a great many were developed. Quinine is still used for the emergency treatment of severe malaria, but it is not a cure because it suppresses the parasite without eliminating it from the body. Nor does it prevent infection.

Another treatment for malaria, used in China for 2000 years, is *artemisin* or artemether, extracted from the wormwood-like plant *Artemisia annua*. The Chinese have led the world in exploiting the medicinal properties of plant products, and there are more to come. For example, there are recent reports of an anti-HIV drug from plants.

Yoghurt
The bio-yoghurts, containing lactobacilli and bifidobacteria (which swarm in the colon of breastfed babies), are other examples of natural therapy (see also page 139, Chapter 7).

Maggots
The larvae of greenbottle flies (maggots) can be useful in treating chronically infected wounds, and over the past three years producers in the UK have supplied 3500 containers of sterile maggots to hundreds of different countries. The maggots eat all dead and infected material, leaving clean, living tissue that is now able to heal itself.

Plant products
Finally, there are one or two promising plant products being developed and assessed right now. These include *teatree oil*, which is active against a wide

range of microbes, although too toxic for other than external use. There are also reports of interesting antimicrobial activity in garlic and cranberry juice.

THOUGHTS ON THE VERY DISTANT FUTURE

I cannot resist final speculation about the future of infectious diseases. This is how it looks to me a hundred or two years from now. As the billions of human beings occupy every corner of the planet and monopolize food supplies, most animal species are doomed to extinction. We will, of course, always keep a small range of domestic animals, but the rich variety of animal life, which we take for granted at present, will be a thing of the past, except for selected species in zoos and wildlife reserves. This means extinction for countless microbial parasites of animals and also extinction for the insects, and ticks that live on these animals.

If this is so, then the only hope of long-term survival for these particular parasites is to switch to the human host. The human body will be almost the last refuge.

But it is not a simple matter. Only a few parasites will be able to make the changes needed for adapting to the human host. Furthermore, if the parasite does much damage, 21st century medical science will pounce on it with vaccines and antimicrobial drugs and eliminate it. A damaging parasite may enjoy temporary success, especially if transmitted by droplets, and may cause much suffering, but its days will be numbered.

Within 50 years, possibly earlier, we will have put an end to nearly all of today's harmful infections. They will be unthinkable in a hygienic, uncontaminated world. The human body will be cleaned up, relieved of its ancient burden of infectious disease, and smallpox will turn out to be the first of a long line of have-beens. Those still tolerated in our species will do little or no harm, either lying low or causing mild hit-and-run infections. It will not be necessary for them to go so far as to attach themselves to our DNA and reach the state of perfect parasitism described for the endogenous retroviruses in Chapter 1, but as far as microbial parasites go, the meek will inherit the earth.

A promising novel strategy, from the microbe's point of view, would be to get humans to look after and encourage the spreading of the infection. Supposing the microbe, in exchange for board and lodging, supplied something humans really value. This is what is referred to as *bribery* in Chapter 6. For instance, one of the herpesviruses transmitted by kissing might make a molecule that caused chronic euphoria, a molecule which did not have the problems associated with heroin and other drugs, and was difficult for humans to synthesize. Would this virus, as long as it did no harm, then be enthusiastically transmitted by the human host? Could it become a welcome guest for pleasure-seeking people, a true mutualist or symbiont with an assured future rather than an old-fashioned parasite?

SELECTED READING

I can find no popular texts on the general subject of infectious diseases, although there is no shortage of action-packed books about dramatic plagues and epidemics. There are only one or two on immunology, but the following will take the reader further into the subject, with fuller accounts and additional details. Most of the sources for this book, however, were technical papers in scientific journals.

Dancer, S. (1999) Mopping up hospital infection. *Br Journal of Hospital Medicine* 43, 85–100. (A reminder about old-fashioned clean liners in hospitals.)

Dixon, B. (1994) *Power Unseen. How microbes rule the world.* WH Freeman, Oxford. (A popular account of microbial life, in the form of 74 vignettes, by an expert communicator.)

Fenner, F. (1982) A successful eradication campaign. Global eradication of smallpox. *Reviews of Infectious Disease*, Vol 4, 916. University of Chicago Press, Chicago. (Description of a major achievement.)

Glendenning, L. (1942) *Source Book of Medical History.* Dover Publications, New York. (A collection of classic descriptions of diseases and remedies, from the Ancient Egyptians to modern times.)

Harper, D. R., Meyer, A. S. (1999) *Men, Mice and Microbes.* Academic Press, London. (A well-written account, focusing on hantaviruses.)

McNeill, William H. (1977) *Plagues and Peoples.* Blackwell, Oxford. (A fascinating, authoritative account of infectious disease in human history.)

Mims, C. A., Nash, A., Stephen, J. (2000) *Mims' Pathogenesis of Infectious Disease.* 5th Edition. Academic Press, London. (An easy-to-read account, for students, of the way microbes cause disease.)

Mims, C. A., Playfair, J. H. L., Roitt, I. M., Wakelin, D., Williams, R. (1998) *Medical Microbiology*. 2nd Edition. Mosby, London. (A straightforward, medical student text.)

Staines, N. A., Brostoff, J., James, K. (1993) *Introducing Immunology*. 2nd Edition. Mosby, London. (A short, basic text.)

Wills, C. (1996) *Plagues. Their Origins, History, and Future*. HarperCollins, New York. (An excellent account of the more dramatic infectious diseases.)

GLOSSARY

Adenoviruses
A group of large DNA viruses. The group itself is also large, with 47 different ones infecting humans. They are very versatile, causing sore throats, conjunctivitis, pneumonia, intestinal illness, and they invade lymphoid tissues. Adenoviruses were discovered when scientists took freshly removed tonsils and adenoids (Greek, *adenos* = gland), grew cells from them in test tubes, and noticed that the cells became sick. This was because a virus was present. In the body, restrained by immune defences, it was present only in an occasional cell, but when the cells were taken into the laboratory and spread out on glass it was free to grow. A large proportion of normal tonsils and adenoids contain adenoviruses.

Adjuvant
A material that enhances the immune response to an antigen, without itself being the antigen.

Amino acid
A basic building block of protein; 20 different ones occur commonly.

Anaerobes
Bacteria (e.g. *tetanus bacilli*) that grow best in the absence of oxygen. Some of them are actually poisoned by oxygen.

Anthrax
A disease due to infection with spores of anthrax bacteria. If the site of initial infection is the skin a swollen, blood-stained blister appears and turns

black (Greek, *anthracis* = coal). Powerful toxins are formed and when untreated the disease can be fatal. When the spores are inhaled into the lungs mortality approaches 100% and this type of anthrax is a weapon in biological warfare.

Antibody (Immunoglobulin = Ig)
A large molecule formed in the *body* during immune response, reacting with antigen on a lock-and-key basis. There are four main types or classes of antibody, IgG, IgM, IgA, IgE.

Antigen
A substance (generally a peptide fragment of a protein) that calls forth an immune response to itself.

Apoptosis
The self-destruction, or suicide, of cells. Of widespread occurrence, as in the development of lymphocytes in the thymus, the disappearance of the tad-pole's tail, or the shrinking of the human embryo's tail to a curled vestige behind the anus.

Arenaviruses
A group of about 12 viruses, for the most part restricted to Africa and South America, each infecting a special species of rodent. In the rodent the infection stays for life and is harmless, but when it spreads to humans it can cause severe disease, as in Lassa fever, South American haemorrhagic fevers, and LCM.

Atom
The units of which molecules are made up; e.g. silver (Ag), sulphur (S). Contain protons, neutrons, electrons.

Autoimmunity
Immunity directed against the body's own tissues; can cause disease (e.g. multiple sclerosis, rheumatoid arthritis).

B cells (B lymphocytes)
The population of lymphocytes derived from Bone-marrow; turn into antibody-producing cells.

Base

A basic chemical compound that combines with acids to form salts. Bases containing nitrogen (e.g. adenine, thymine) are the building blocks of DNA and RNA.

BCG

The Bacillus Calmette–Guérin, developed by the French scientists Albert Calmette and Camille Guérin. They took a strain of tuberculosis from cattle and grew it in artificial culture in the laboratory for more than ten years (1908–1918), until it no longer caused disease. This is the vaccine, and each dose contains at least a million living bacteria, which multiply at the site of injection into the arm and in nearby lymph nodes to give lasting immunity. It is used throughout the world to immunize children against tuberculosis, and more people alive today have had BCG than have had any other vaccine.

Bone marrow

The soft core of bones, well supplied with blood vessels, site of production of red and white blood cells.

Botulism

This neurological disease is due to a toxin formed by *Clostridium botulinum*, a free-living bacterium that can contaminate meat or vegetables. In 1793 a large sausage (Latin, *botulus* = sausage) was eaten by 13 people in Wildbad, Germany, making them all ill; six died. A mere gram of the toxin is enough to kill ten million mice.

Brucellosis

A bacterial infection of cows, pigs and goats, causing chronic illness when it spreads to humans.

Candida

A fungus, present on skin and in the mouth and intestine of most people, in the form of a single-celled yeast. A distant relative of brewer's yeast. Normally kept under control by CMI. Can cause thrush, with white patches (Latin, *candidus* = white) inside the mouth, or vaginal thrush with irritation and discharge. In those with serious immune defects the yeast sends out long branches, as if foraging, which enable it to penetrate tissues, invade the blood, and cause life-threatening infection.

Capillary
The smallest blood vessel, visible only under the microscope.

Chemotaxis
The moving of a cell towards (or away from) a chemical substance.

Cilia
Fine, firmly anchored hairs protruding from cells, moving backwards and forwards with a regular beat. On a sheet of cells the beat of the cilia is co-ordinated and moves liquids across the surface. Under the microscope it looks like the movement on the surface of a wheatfield in a gentle breeze.

CMI (cell-mediated immunity)
Immunity expressed by cells, especially T cells and macrophages.

Coagulase
This enzyme released by invading staphylococci causes blood plasma to coagulate and form a layer round the bacteria, interfering with access of white blood cells.

Complement
A group of about 30 proteins present in blood, forming a powerful defence system. The principal proteins are sequentially activated (converted into active form) when antigen combines with antibody. They cause inflammation and play a vital part in phagocytosis, opsonization and chemotaxis.

Corneal
To do with the cornea, the transparent outer layer of the eye under the conjunctiva.

Corynebacterium diphtheriae
Diphtheria bacterium. *Koryne* (Greek = club) refers to the club-like shape of the bacteria.

Coxsackie viruses
There are 26 different types. Most infect via the intestine, and they can cause meningitis and throat ulcers. Others cause myositis (inflammation of muscle) and heart attacks (inflammation of heart muscle).

Cyst

A special form of a protozoan parasite, analogous to the bacterial spore, that is resistant to drying, heat, etc., and adapted for the hazardous journey from host to host. Formed by toxoplasma, giardia and amoebic dysentery parasites. Also, a special form of parasitic worm, covered with a thick, resistant wall, as in the case of the hydatid cyst, the form of the dog tapeworm in human tissues.

Cytokines

The hormones of the immune system. There are at least 20 different ones, including interferons and interleukins. They act as the language by which immune cells speak to one another, usually in brief and local pulses. When present in excessive amounts they can have harmful effects.

Cytomegalovirus

A large virus and a well-behaved one. In a child it is harmless but if a woman gets her first infection during pregnancy it can invade the placenta and the fetus and interfere with organ development (like rubella and syphilis).

Delayed hypersensitivity

A reaction of redness and swelling, not visible until 1–2 days after introducing an antigen into the skin of a sensitized individual. An expression of CMI.

Diarrhoea

Generally defined as the passage of liquid faeces, but the best definition, perhaps, is the passage of faeces that takes the shape of the receptacle rather than has its own shape. It can be regarded on the one hand as a microbial device for spreading the infection, or on the other as a host defence to hasten the expulsion of the offending microbe.

DNA (deoxyribonucleic acid)

The chemical substance that genes are made of. The DNA molecule is a long one, made up of different bases as building blocks, acting as the conveyer of hereditary information. Each gene consists of a coded tape, analogous to the bar code on supermarket items, with a unique sequence of bases that give it the capacity to form (code for) a particular protein.

Dysentery

A severe diarrhoeal disease with blood and mucus. Can be due to bacteria

(*Shigella*) or to amoebae. The amoebae (*Entamoeba histolytica*) are common in tropical and subtropical countries; they are ingested in the form of resistant cysts. After contact with stomach acid the growing forms of the amoebae are released and these multiply, causing dysentery. Fresh cysts are produced and shed in faeces.

EB virus (Epstein–Barr virus)
Discovered in 1964 in Bristol, England. It is a herpesvirus, the group of viruses present throughout the world that includes herpes simplex (cold sore) virus and varicella zoster (chickenpox-shingles) virus. EB virus is transmitted by saliva, grows in epithelial cells and in B cells, causes glandular fever, and then remains in the body in latent form.

Endemic
Something that is present in a geographical area or population, and remains there without being reintroduced from outside.

Endothelium
A sheet of flattened cells lining a blood or lymph vessel, or the heart.

Enzymes
Protein molecules that promote chemical reactions without taking part in them. Microbes have many enzymes essential for their metabolism and multiplication.

Epithelium
A sheet of cells covering a surface of the body, including the skin, the lining of the intestinal, respiratory and urogenital tracts.

Escherichia coli
An intestinal resident, one of the normal flora. There are dozens of different varieties of *E. coli*, each with different antigens and a different ability to cause trouble. Traveller's diarrhoea is most commonly due to an encounter with a new type of *E. coli*.

Filariasis
A disease due to parasitic worms, spread by mosquitoes. The adult worm lives in the lymphatic system of e.g. the lower leg, blocking the lymphatic drainage of fluid, resulting in chronic swelling (elephantiasis) of leg. It produces microscopic larvae that enter blood and are taken up by mosquitoes.

Food-poisoning
Illness coming on a day or two after eating food containing microbes or microbial toxins.

Ganglion
A knot-like swelling (Greek, *ganglion* = a swelling), a mass of nerve cells. Sensory ganglia supply sensation to the skin, and are present on each side of the spinal cord and at the base of the brain.

Gas gangrene
Bacterial infection of a wound, involving muscles, with destruction and gas formation.

Genome
The genetic equipment of a living creature. Consists of DNA, but in the case of viruses can be either DNA or RNA.

Giardia
A protozoan parasite causing diarrhoea. Present in the intestines of many animals, and its cysts contaminate rivers, drinking water.

Gonorrhoea
Sexually transmitted disease (STD) caused by the bacterium *Neisseria gonorrhoeae*, of which there are many strains. The bacteria infect the urethra and vagina (or rectum, throat, conjunctiva), causing a white discharge. The male experiences great discomfort on urination and the disease was aptly called 'chaude pisse' in 14th century France. Infection is often asymptomatic in females, and sometimes in males. Occasionally other urogenital organs are invaded (e.g. Fallopian tubes). As with many other STDs, males infect females more easily than females infect males.

Haemophilus influenzae
A bacterium, so-called because it was once thought to be the cause of influenza. It colonizes the nose and throat, from where it can spread into the body, especially in children, and give rise to pneumonia or meningitis. Responsible for more than half a million deaths each year. In developing countries one in three children carry the bacterium in their nose and throat; only a tenth as many in industrialized countries. An excellent vaccine (Hib) is available, which consists of the bacterial outer coat or capsule (a type of sugar called a polysaccharide), attached to a protein to make it more effective.

Helminths (worms)
These are unlike other parasites insofar as each individual is made up of many cells (multicellular). Some (e.g. threadworms) are almost universal human companions. Their life cycle may require more than one host species, such as a sheep plus a dog for the tapeworm of hydatid disease. Humans with schistosomiasis or dogs with tapeworms are infected with single worms, which stay as one worm although they may liberate thousands of eggs. Hence a heavy level of infection requires a large invasion or repeated invasions. A virus or bacterium, in contrast, achieves a heavy infection simply by multiplying in the human host.

Histamine
A substance formed by mast cells, causing dilation of blood vessels, increased acid secretion in the stomach, and other 'allergic' effects.

HLA: see MHC

Immunoglobulins (Ig = antibodies)
Globular-shaped proteins. Often called gammaglobulins because they are in the 'gamma' part of serum after it has been electrophoresed.

Incubation period
The period between getting infected and showing signs of disease.

Interferons
Interferons alpha and beta are antiviral substances produced by infected cells, preventing infection of neighbouring cells. Interferon gamma is a cytokine formed by immune cells.

Interleukin (Il)
A type of cytokine that carries vital signals between immune cells. Il-2 is a basic driving force for T cells needed for their proliferation. There are about 18 different interleukins.

Lactobacilli
Lactic acid-producing bacteria, normal residents of vagina.

LCM (lymphocytic choriomeningitis)
A naturally occurring and lifelong virus infection of mice and hamsters. Does not harm the cells it grows in and illness in the experimentally

infected natural host is due to the immune response. Infected humans may develop meningitis.

Legionnaires' disease
A lung infection caused by inhalation of the free-living bacterium *Legionnella pneumophila*, after it has colonized air-conditioning systems, water-cooling towers, etc., and become airborne. Can cause a fatal pneumonia.

Leptospirosis
A bacterial infection of dogs, rats, etc. Human infection follows exposure to urine of infected animal, for instance immersion in water of a rat-infested canal. About 50 cases a year in the UK.

Listeria
Bacteria widely distributed in nature, present in plants, farm animals, etc. Humans are infected from cow's milk, vegetables. Can cause severe disease in pregnant women, newborn infants and elderly people.

Lyme disease
A disease named after the town in Connecticut, USA, where the first cases were recognized in 1975. Caused by the bacterium *Borrelia burgdorferi*, and occurs in USA, parts of Europe and elsewhere. The bacteria infect deer and mice, and are spread by their ticks, sometimes to humans. Twelve thousand Americans developed Lyme disease in 1995.

Lymph
The colourless fluid, containing immune cells, that passes from tissues to lymph nodes and thence to the blood.

Lymph vessels
Channels carrying lymph from the tissues to lymph nodes, and then back to the blood.

Lymphocyte
A cell from the lymphoid system, present in lymph and blood as a type of white cell. B lymphocytes are distinguished from T lymphocytes.

Lymphoid system
This refers to the total mass of immune cells (lymphocytes, macrophages, etc.) in the body. If all were in one piece it would be the size of a football.

Lysosome
The sac present inside phagocytes, containing defensive substances, enzymes, etc.

Macrophage
A large phagocyte in tissues and in blood; longer lived than polymorph phagocyte.

Malaria (Plasmodium)
Four different species infect humans; most harmful is *Plasmodium falciparum*. Malaria kills more than a million people each year. The parasite, introduced by mosquito, first infects liver cells, where it can lie low for long periods, and it then invades red blood cells. In the acute disease fever occurs every 2–3 days as fresh sets of red cells are infected and destroyed. Long-term effects are anaemia and chronic ill health. A special form of parasite is produced in blood for uptake by biting mosquitoes, growing in their salivary glands.

Mast cell
A cell found especially in respiratory and intestinal tracts, to which IgE antibodies attach and which releases histamine and other substances.

MHC (Major Histocompatibility Complex) or HLA (Human Leucocyte Antigen) in humans
These are the molecules present on the surface of all cells in the case of class 1 MHC, or only on certain immune cells (class 2 MHC). They give the cells of each individual a unique label, identical twins having the same set. Grafts from one individual to an unrelated one are rejected because the foreign MHC molecules are recognized by the immune system. Their function is to display antigens on the cell surface, either to start off the immune response (class 2 MHC) or to tell cytotoxic T lymphocytes that the cell is infected (class 1 MHC). Different MHC molecules prefer to take on board different peptide antigens, and to cope with the vast range of peptides from microbes it is best to have as wide a range of MHC molecules as possible. Greater variety in MHC genes of humans ensures that there will always be a few of us who can resist any terrible new disease that arises. Too much variation, however, gives the immune system a trigger-happy sensitivity that can lead to autoimmunity ('friendly fire'). A suitable balance is needed.

Milk
Contains many things that protect the infant against infection, including

IgA antibodies and lysosome (see Glossary). Colostrum, the first milk that comes after childbirth, is especially rich in IgA antibodies.

Molecule
The smallest unit of a substance, made up of different atoms. Can be very small, such as a molecule of water (H_2O with three atoms) or of table salt (NaCl with two atoms), or very large such as proteins and DNA, consisting of thousands of atoms.

Monkeypox
An infection of monkeys in Central Africa, caused by a virus closely related to smallpox. Humans in close contact with monkeys have been infected, suffering a smallpox-like disease, but it fails to spread through more than a few person-to-person transfers.

Monoclonal antibody
The antibody formed by a clone of B cells (derived from a single parent cell), of a particular class and reacting with a particular antigen.

Mumps
A disease caused by a virus related to measles. Spreads by saliva and droplets, invading salivary glands, occasionally the coverings of the brain (meningitis) or various other glands (testis, mammary gland, pancreas). The classical victim has a swollen and tender parotid gland at the side of the face. Excellent vaccine available.

Mutation
A change in DNA, generally small. Most mutations are harmful and the microbe carrying it is eliminated. If the mutation is advantageous it tends to spread in the population and replace the original form.

NK cell (natural killer cell)
A type of T cell operating as part of the early defence system, within the first day or two of infection. Unlike other T cells, the NK cell does not recognize individual antigens but kills cells that are not displaying MHC class 1 labels, because these are usually infected by viruses.

Node (lymph node = lymph gland)
A visible, rounded collection of lymphoid and other immune cells. Has its own supply of blood and lymph.

Glossary

Opportunists
Microbes that are normally harmless but take opportunities and cause damage when host defences are weakened.

Opsonin
A substance, usually antibody, that combines with the surface of a microbe and makes it more easily phagocytosed.

Oxygen radicals
A type of oxygen formed by phagocytes, with potent activity against microbes. Also capable of damaging host tissues.

Parainfluenza viruses
Related to influenza viruses, these cause common cold, bronchitis, croup, pneumonia, especially in children. Four types.

Pasteurization
A mild heat treatment (63–65°C) that kills disease-causing microbes without spoiling taste or quality of foods like milk, cheese and beer. Developed by Louis Pasteur (1822–1895).

Pathogen
A disease-causing microbe.

Peptide
Part of a protein; a substance made up of two or more amino acids.

Peritoneal, pleural cavities
Potential cavities rather than real ones, surrounding the organs of the abdomen and chest, lined by a continuous sheet of living cells and containing macrophages.

Persistent virus
A virus that stays in the body for long periods after infection, often for life, e.g. most herpesviruses, or LCM virus in mice.

pH
A numerical method of expressing acidity or alkalinity. Pure water is 'neutral' (pH 7.0), acids have pH less than 7.0 and alkalis greater than 7.0. It is a logarithmic scale, so that pH 5.0 is ten times as acidic as pH 6.0. Stomach pH is about 3.0.

Placebo (Latin = I will please)
Supposedly inactive material given to patient, whose response is compared with that seen in those given the substance being tested. Placebo effect: healing effect caused by the placebo on its own. In certain diseases the beneficial effect of the placebo can be considerable, because of the feeling that something is being done, something magical perhaps.

Plasma
The clear, slightly straw-coloured fluid that remains when the red and white cells are removed from unclotted blood.

Plasmid
A small piece of DNA (containing up to 100 genes) in a bacterium, but not part of the bacterial chromosome (containing most of the DNA) and replicating independently.

Pneumococcus
Streptococcus pneumoniae, the commonest cause of bacterial pneumonia. Often responsible for death in the elderly ('the old man's friend'), but occurs also in the young and healthy. Can cause meningitis, and is becoming resistant to penicillin and other antibiotics. Luckily only 23 of the 84 different types commonly cause disease, and the vaccine takes care of these types.

Pneumocystis carinii
Almost universal fungal parasite of human lung. Only causes disease when immune defences impaired.

Polymorph
Polymorphonuclear white cell: Metchnikov's 'microphage'; short-lived phagocyte, abundant in blood and inflamed tissues; originates in bone marrow.

Polyomaviruses
So-called because the sort found in mice cause many types of tumour, hence poly (many) + oma (tumour). Human variety spread mostly by droplets and reach the kidneys, grow in cells lining the urinary channels and are excreted for a while in urine. They cause no damage and tend to go latent (see page 186), but reactivate and reappear in urine during pregnancy, or when immune responses are defective.

Poxviruses

A group of large DNA viruses causing skin lesions (pocks); e.g. mousepox, goatpox, monkeypox, smallpox and myxoma virus (in rabbits).

Prions

PRoteinaceous INfectious agents; the smallest replicating agents, causing scrapie (sheep), BSE (cattle), and CJD and kuru (humans). Highly resistant to heat, disinfectants, etc.

Proteins

Large molecules made up of hundreds of different amino acids. Proteins form the basic structure of cells and enzymes, and play a fundamental role in life (Greek, *proteus* = primary).

Psittacosis

A lung infection caused by the bacterium *Chlamydia psittaci*; acquired by inhaling dust from infected parrots (psittacines) and other birds.

Relapsing fever

A disease caused by *Borrelia recurrentis*, a spiral-shaped bacterium, with episodes of fever (hence relapsing). Transmitted by ticks or lice. A related bacterium (*B. burgdorferi*) causes Lyme disease, transferred to humans in the USA and parts of Europe by ticks from deer and mice.

Rheumatic fever

Inflammation of the heart caused when a person forms antibodies to streptococci that also react (cross-react) with the heart. Repeated attacks by different strains of streptococci can damage valves of the heart. The disease is still common, with 370,000 new cases each year in parts of the world with poor access to medical care and antibiotics.

RNA (ribonucleic acid)

The intermediate substance through which DNA makes proteins and thus creates living material. The instructions coded on the DNA tape are transformed into RNA, which then constructs and assembles the protein.

Roundworm (Ascaris lumbricoides)

Large (20–30 cm long) white worm; lives for six months to three years in the human intestine, the female laying a quarter of a million eggs a day. Eggs find their way into the mouth of others, hatch to form larvae, which migrate through the body and cause allergic reactions before settling down for good in the intestine. Occurs worldwide but commonest in tropical and subtropical countries.

Rubella
Or German measles; is a virus infection that is usually so mild that it is not noticed. The tragic effects are seen when it infects pregnant women. They themselves are unaffected, but as the virus spreads through the body it infects the placenta and reaches the fetus (like cytomegalovirus and syphilis). If this occurs early in pregnancy it interferes with organ development and the newborn baby may suffer from heart disease, eye or ear defects, mental retardation.

Salmonella
A group of rod-shaped bacteria. *Salmonella typhi* causes the disease typhoid, other *Salmonella* (hundreds of different types) infect the intestines of animals and birds and can cause food-poisoning (salmonellosis) in humans.

Scarlet fever
A disease presenting with a red rash, and due to *Streptococcus pyogenes*. The rash is caused by a toxin from the bacteria.

Schistosomiasis
A disease common in parts of Africa (200 million people infected), caused by a fluke (a type of worm). Larvae from infected snails enter water and then penetrate human skin. Heavy infection causes chronic ill health, with urinary symptoms (blood in urine) and excretion of parasite in urine, enlarged liver and spleen.

Septicaemia (blood-poisoning)
The presence of multiplying bacteria in the blood, causing severe illness.

Serum
The clear, slightly straw-coloured fluid that separates out when blood is clotted.

Shigella
Bacteria infecting the intestine of humans. Cause of bacilliary dysentery.

SSPE (Subacute Sclerosing PanEncephalitis)
A very rare complication of measles. The virus reaches the brain and slowly multiplies, causing fatal encephalitis after about ten years.

Staphylococci
Spherical bacteria, forming grape-like clusters when they grow (Greek, *staphylos* = grape, *coccos* = berry); include *Staphylococcus epidermidis*, the skin resident, and *S. aureus* which can cause boils, abscesses, septicaemia, etc. Antibiotics, washing machines and soap have made such things memories.

Sterility
The absence of living, multiplying microbes.

Streptococci
Spherical bacteria, forming chains when they grow (Greek, *streptos* = chain, *coccos* = berry); include both residents and pathogens. *Streptococcus pyogenes* causes sore throats, scarlet fever and other severe diseases, and *S. pneumoniae* causes pneumonia.

T cells (T lymphocytes)
A population of lymphocytes whose development depends on the presence of the thymus gland; responsible for CMI. Subdivided into helper and cytotoxic T cells.

Thymus
An organ lying in the front of the chest (the sweetbread). Very active in early life, a lymphocyte production unit where the product is carefully checked and those reacting with 'self' are eliminated.

Tissue
The cellular network of which the body is made up, as opposed to the separate structures or organs. Hence muscle tissue, nervous tissue, connective tissue, etc.

Toxin
A poisonous substance produced by a microbe (e.g. tetanus toxin).

Toxoid
A toxin that has been treated by heat or formalin so that it is no longer

poisonous but is still able to cause the formation of antibody that neutralizes the toxin (e.g. tetanus toxoid).

Toxoplasma
A protozoan parasite of the domestic cat, infecting its intestine and present as cysts in cat faeces. Oral infection of humans normally causes only mild disease but it can be more serious when it reaches the fetus or infects a person with a weakened immune response.

Trachoma
The most famous eye infection in history, causing eventual blindness. Due to the bacterium *Chlamydia trachomatis*, and spread by fingers, flies, towels, etc.

Tract
Alimentary, respiratory or urinogenital tract. Refers to the canals lining these parts of the body, conveying liquids, gases, nutrients, waste products.

Tuberculin
A mixture of antigens from tuberculosis bacteria, introduced into the skin to test for delayed hypersensitivity to the bacteria.

Typhus
A disease caused by *Rickettsia prowazeki*, transmitted by the human body louse. Disease thrives when lice thrive, that is to say when clothes and bodies are rarely washed, for instance due to poverty or war.

Urinary infection
Infection of the urinary tract. It generally takes place by way of the urethra to the bladder (cystitis), and occasionally spreads from here up the ureters to the kidney (nephritis).

Vessel
A channel (e.g. artery, vein, lymphatic) through which blood or lymph flows.

INDEX

Index